Applied Science and Pathology OSCEs In Surgery

Zakk Borton BMBS BMedSci (Hons) MRCS

Charles Handford MBChB (Hons) MRCS DMCC

Alexander Logan MBChB MSc MRCS PGCME

© 2017 MD+ Publishing

Published by: MD+ Publishing

Cover Design: Alexander Logan

ISBN-10: 0993113877

ISBN-13: 978-0993113871

Printed in the United Kingdom

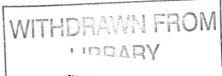

D1583793

CONTENTS

Contributors

Preface

Chapter 1: Applied Science

Chapter 2: Pathology

Contributors

Laura Beddard MBChB MRCS
ST3 T&O Registrar
Wessex Deanery

Yan Mei Goh MBChB PG Dip Clin Ed MRCS
Core Surgical Trainee
North West Deanery

Yan Li Goh MBChB PG Dip Clin Ed MRCS
General Surgery Research Registrar
North West Deanery

Jeremy Wilson
Consultant Colorectal Surgeon
Wirral University Teaching Hospitals
NHS Foundation Trust

Selina Graham MBChB MRCS
Core Surgical Trainee
Severn Deanery

James Davis MBChB MRCS
Core Surgical Trainee

Yasmin Grant MBChB MRCS
Core Surgical Trainee

Simon McLuney MBChB MRCS
Core Surgical Trainee

Sanjeet Singh Avtaar Singh MBChB (Edin), MSc (Edin), MRCSEd
Core Surgical Trainee
NHS Scotland

Raymond Rueben MBChB
ST1 Radiology
NHS Greater Glasgow And Clyde

Sit Lee Euan MBChB (Edin)
Clinical Teaching Fellow in Diabetics
and Endocrinology
NHS Ayrshire and Arran

Laura Henderson BSc MBChB MRCS
Core Surgical Trainee
West Midlands Deanery

Habib Tafazal, BSc MBChB FRCS
Warwick Hospital
West Midlands Deanery

Gaural Patel MSc MRCS
Core Surgical Trainee
Wales Deanery

Nazan Can Guru Naidu MRCS DOHNS
Chase Farm and Barnet Hospital
Royal Free Trust Hospitals
London Deanery

Preface

The authors and editors of this text are all surgeons at various stages of their careers who have successfully attained their membership of the Royal College of Surgeons.

The most useful way to prepare for the MRCS Part B is by testing your knowldge and working in pairs to simulate the real exam.

This book draws on the authors' collective experience of both sitting the exam and teaching others and uses realistic scenarios as have appeared in the actual exam.

The text can be used alone to test your knowledge but works best when used to test colleagues.

Good Luck.

1 APPLIED SCIENCES

1.1 Burns

Scenario

A 34-year-old man is brought in as a trauma call after being found in a burning house. Part of the building collapsed and hit his right arm before he was trapped for approximately 5 minutes in an enclosed space.

How would you initially assess this patient?

This patient needs to be assessed along ATLS principles. His C-spine should be protected with triple immobilisation until it can be cleared clinically or radiologically. An airway assessment requires particular attention to potential progression of oedema and in some cases early intubation may be indicated. High flow oxygen should be applied. His breathing assessment includes observation for burns affecting his chest wall that may impede ventilation, especially circumferential burns. Oxygen saturations and oxygen requirements should be noted and the chest percussed and auscultated. IV access with two large bore cannulas is required, with blood taken for FBC, U&E, LFTs, CK and group and save. A venous blood gas should also be performed. IV fluid resuscitation should be started. Heart rate and blood pressure should be recorded, and the heart auscultated. Disability should be assessed with GCS or the more simple AVPU scoring system. Full exposure is vital in order to calculate the area affected by burns and stop the burning process, however ensure the patient is kept warm to prevent hypothermia. Note that clothing adherent to the skin should not be ripped away in resus.

What features would concern you that his airway may be compromised?

In this history of being in an enclosed space there would be a risk of airway compromise. Other important points to note would be soot around the nostrils, singed facial hair, facial burns, hoarse voice, cough or hypoxia.

What method could you use to calculate the percentage surface area affected by the burns?

The rule of 9's divides the body into areas of 9%. This allows a quick estimate of the area affected. The palm of the patient represents 1% of TBSA and this can also be used to calculate the area affected.
The Lund and Browner Burn chart is the most accurate method and is widely available; there are specific charts available for children.
It is important to note areas of erythema only are not included in the burn area calculation.

How do you clinically differentiate between the depth of the burn?

• Epidermal (first degree) burns are erythematic and painful; usually there are no blisters. The skin is in tact. Capillary refill time will be rapid.
• Partial thickness burns can be split into superficial and deep (second degree). They are red/mottled in appearance. Blister formation and swelling will occur. Painful and hypersensitive. Capillary refill will be present but slower than in first-degree burns and will decrease in response as burn deepens.
• Full thickness (third degree) burns are dry, dark, white or charred in appearance. There will be no capillary refill/blanching and pain will be absent.

How would you establish the volume of fluid replacement required?

Prediction of requirement in the first 24 hours can be achieved using the Parkland formula:
- Fluid Requirements = TBSA burned (%) x Weight (kg) x 2-4mL
- Half Is given over 8 hours and the remaining half over 16 hours

It is important to remember this is a guide and physiological parameters should be measured. Urinary catheterisation is required. If the patient is in shock standard resuscitation principles must be applied (i.e. fluid boluses).

How would you monitor response to fluid resuscitation?

Patients require a urinary catheter, as urinary output is a sensitive marker of fluid status. This should be greater than 0.5ml/kg/hour in adults. Other markers that need monitoring are skin turgor, pulse, blood pressure and capillary refill time. If monitoring is difficult or a large volume of fluid is required a central venous line may also be required.

What first aid management would you apply to the burns?

Burns need covering in order to reduce insensible fluid losses, prevent hypothermia and reduce infection risk. Laying (not circumferential wrapping) cling film on the wound is commonly used. Some utilise antimicrobial ointments and light dressings however these must only be used after assessment by a burns specialist as the ointment can make subsequent assessment of depth/severity challenging. Clinical photography in all burns is a useful tool.

The patient is found to have 25% partial thickness burn affecting the left arm, chest and abdomen. During the time he is in ED he becomes wheezy and his oxygen saturations decrease to 94% despite being on 15L O2.

How would you now manage the patient?

He requires re-assessment along ATLS principles. His airway has now become a concern, and the anaesthetic team should be informed. He now requires intubation and mechanical ventilation. Breathing and circulation also need to be re-assessed and treatment started.

The patient is intubated in ED and taken to ITU for ventilatory support. The oxygen saturations increase back to 98%. The blood pressure is now 84/68 and urine output for the previous hour is 20ml. They have received 2L of the 4.5L required in the first 8 hours.

How would you manage the circulatory system?

Other parameters as outlined above, such as skin turgor and capillary refill time should be assessed. The patient requires a fluid bolus of 500ml administered immediately. The response to this can be measured by blood pressure and urine output. If they fail to respond to fluid resuscitation, inotropic or vasopressor support may be required.

Where should this patient ultimately be managed?

This patient meets the criteria for transfer to a specialist burns centre due to over 25% TBSA with inhalation injury.

What additional treatment/intervention may be required when he reaches the burns unit?

Escharotomy of the burns affecting the chest wall may be required if chest wall movement is reduced and therefore ventilation is compromised. If the burn of his left arm is circumferential eschartomy may be required to preserve distal blood flow.

Bronchoscopy may well be performed by the intensive care team.

What other criteria are there for transfer to the specialist burns unit?

The suggested minimum threshold for referral into specialised burn care services can be summarised as:
o All burns ≥2% TBSA in children or ≥3% in adults
o All full thickness burns
o All circumferential burns
o Any burn not healed in 2 weeks
o Any burn with suspicion of non-accidental injury should be referred to a Burn Unit/Centre for expert assessment within 24 hours

In addition, the following factors should prompt a discussion with a Consultant in a specialised burn care service and consideration given to referral:
o All burns to hands, feet, face, perineum or genitalia
o Any chemical, electrical or friction burn
o Any cold injury
o Any unwell/febrile child with a burn
o Any concerns regarding burn injuries and co-morbidities that may affect treatment or healing of the burn
o If the above criteria/threshold is not met then continue with local care and dressings as required
o If burn wound changes in appearance / signs of infection or there are concerns regarding healing then discuss with a specialised burn service
o If there is any suspicion of Toxic shock syndrome (TSS) then refer early

The patient is transferred to the burns unit and an escharotomy is performed.

What early complications can arise in patients with severe burns?

Burns may become secondarily infected. However the use of prophylactic antibiotics is not routine. Fluid losses can result in acute kidney injury and hyperkalaemia requiring haemodialysis. This is best prevented with early fluid resuscitation starting in the ED. Other organs that can be affected include the lungs, which can develop acute respiratory distress syndrome (ARDS) and the gastrointestinal system in the form of peptic ulceration (Curling's ulcer) due to mucosal atrophy secondary to ischaemia. Disseminated intravascular coagulation (DIC) is also associated. The patient will also become profoundly catabolic.

Once the patient's condition has stabilised what surgical options are available for covering the burns?

Split skin grafting is one option, which is most commonly performed in the acute setting to provide coverage to the burn. Their use is restricted to patients who have enough skin that has not been affected by the burns. However large areas can be covered with this type of graft due to meshing of the donor skin. Full thickness grafts give a better cosmetic appearance than split skin grafts and are reserved for areas such as the face and hands. Vascular supply to areas covered with a full thickness graft must be good in order to support the metabolic requirements of the graft. In other circumstances local or free flaps may be used.

APPLIED SCIENCES

How should patients with severe burns receive nutrition?

Metabolic requirements of these patients are high, therefore nutrition is extremely important and enteral feeding is preferred. Early enteral feeding is associated with a reduced incidence of peptic ulceration. Dieticians should be involved in calculating patient's requirements, which will include an increased protein intake. Wound healing will be slowed with inadequate nutrition.

SUMMARY

Burns is often an area of examination as it can be used to assess many areas of knowledge and therefore it is important to have a thorough understanding of the topic from presentation, ITU care and surgical interventions and options.

The "Rule of 9's":
Head and each arm = 9%
Back, chest and abdomen each = 18%
Each leg = 18%
Perineum = 1%
Lund-Browder charts are more accurate and should always be used to calculate BSA in children

Parkland Formula:
Adults:
3-4 ml / kg / % burn of Hartmann's solution
- 50% of volume in first 8 hours and 50% in the next 16 hours
- 1st 50% of volume is given within 8 hours from time of burn
- Above is a guide – titrate to ≥ 0.5ml/kg/hour urine output

Children: As above but add maintenance fluids.

TOP TIPS

 Remember to assess for any inhalation injury. The subsequent odema may necessitate intubation to avoid breathing difficulties.

1.2 | Nutrition

> ## Scenario
>
> A 72 year old man is admitted to the general surgical ward with ischaemic bowel. He is taken to theatre and has a small bowel resection and primary anastomosis. He returns to the high dependency unit (HDU) with a Ryles' tube and IV fluids. Post operative instructions state he should be kept nil by mouth.

What broad types of feeding are there?

Feeding can either be enteral or parenteral.

What is enteral feeding and how can it be given?

Enteral feeding is when nutrition is absorbed from the gastrointestinal tract. This can be when food is taken orally, via a nasogastric tube, nasojejunal tube or a percutaneous endoscopic gastrostomy (PEG).

The patient develops an ileus and enteral feeding is withheld for 6 days following surgery

What is the metabolic response to fasting?

Due to a low level of glucose insulin levels fall and glucagon levels rise. This results in hepatic glycogenolysis. Muscle is broken down to provide amino acids, and these are used in gluconeogenesis. The liver increases its ability to perform lipolysis resulting in ketone body production. The brain switches to uses ketone bodies instead of glucose as its primary energy source. Ultimately the metabolic rate reduces.

What are the disadvantages of using glucose as the main energy source in illness?

People can develop hyperglycaemia and glucose intolerance during the period of being unwell. This means that any excess glucose is converted into lipids in the liver, which can result in fatty liver and derangement of the liver function tests. The respiratory quotient of carbohydrates is higher, so more carbon dioxide is produced which can affect ventilation.

How do the nutritional requirements of a critically ill patient differ from a well person?

Ill patients often have an intolerance of glucose, and therefore less carbohydrate may be given in the diet in an attempt to achieve glycaemic control. A higher proportion of protein is required due to the catabolic state.

Name some of the essential minerals required.

Zinc, copper, chromium and magnesium.

APPLIED SCIENCES

The patient remains in HDU and develops a wound problem. Examination is shown below.

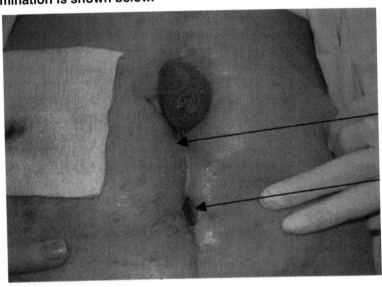

What is the diagnosis?

This patient has a enterocutaneous fistula.

What indications are there for parenteral feeding?

The absolute indication for parenteral nutrition is the presence of an enterocutaneous fistula. Other gastrointestinal diagnoses such as small bowel syndrome or inflammatory bowel disease may also require total parenteral nutrition (TPN). It is also indicated when patients are critically unwell, such as with sepsis, and unlikely to tolerate enteral feeding within seven days.

How is TPN administered?

In most cases TPN is given via a central line due to the high osmolality of the feed causing damage to peripheral vessels. If the feed is diluted in some cases peripheral parenteral nutrition can be given. The line should be dedicated to only TPN reducing the risk of line complications.

What are the complications of parenteral nutrition?

There are complications related to the line and those related to the feed. Central line insertion can result in bleeding and pneumothorax. In the longer term the line can get blocked, it can migrate and become infected. Metabolic complications include hyperglycaemia or hypoglycaemia, electrolyte disturbances and deranged liver function.

What is refeeding syndrome?

It is a complication caused by shifts in fluid and electrolytes after the re-introduction of nutrition. Blood tests show hypophosphataemia, hypokalaemia and mineral deficiencies. Patients develop peripheral oedema as a result of fluid overload. In some cases it can be fatal. Risk of refeeding syndrome is higher in patients with a low BMI, prolonged period of time with little nutrition, unintentional weight loss, existing electrolyte disturbances prior to starting feeding and a history of alcohol abuse.

What blood tests need to be measured when TPN is started?

Capillary blood glucose should be measured throughout the day. Each day renal function and electrolytes should be checked. In addition albumin, calcium, magnesium, phosphate and liver function tests need to be checked.

Blood tests are performed and the results are below:

Na 132 mmol/L   Mg2+ 0.84 mmol/L Albumin 18   Glucose 19.8 mmol/L
K 2.6 mmol/L   Ca2+ 2.34 mmol/L ALP 129 U/L
Ur 6.4 mmol/L   PO4- 0.32 mmol/L ALT 37 U/L
Cr 87 µmol/L   Bili 18 µmol/L

Explain these results

The patient has a low potassium, low phosphate and low albumin with a high glucose. The patient is likely to have refeeding syndrome.

How would you manage a patient with refeeding syndrome?

The rate of feeding should be slowed and potassium and phosphate should be replaced, ideally intravenously. The dieticians should be involved to adjust the composition of the feed.

When should you consider discontinuing TPN?

Parenteral nutrition should be replaced by enteral feeding as soon as possible. Once the proximal small bowel has regained its function and enough nutrition can be absorbed to provide the required nutritional requirements enteral feeding can be started.

SUMMARY

Total parenteral nutrition (TPN) is provided when the gastrointestinal tract is nonfunctional because of an interruption in its continuity (it is blocked, or has a leak - a fistula) or because its absorptive capacity is impaired.

TPN fully bypasses the GI tract and normal methods of nutrient absorption.

In most cases TPN is given via a central line due to the high osmolality of the feed causing damage to peripheral vessels. If the feed is diluted in some cases peripheral parenteral nutrition can be given. The line should be dedicated to only TPN reducing the risk of line complications.

There are complications related to the line and those related to the feed. Central line insertion can result in bleeding and pneumothorax. In the longer term the line can get blocked, it can migrate and become infected. Metabolic complications include hyperglycaemia or hypoglycaemia, electrolyte disturbances and deranged liver function.

APPLIED SCIENCES

TOP TIPS

✚ Prepared solutions generally consist of water and electrolytes; glucose, amino acids, and lipids; essential vitamins, minerals and trace elements are added or given separately.

✚ TPN can also be configured for individual patient needs and this is usually managed by a specialist nurse.

1.3 Pancreatitis

Scenario

A 56 year old alcoholic gentleman presents with a 12 hour history of central abdominal pain and vomiting following a heavy drinking session. The pain is radiating to his back, he is hypotensive and tachycardic.

What is your differential diagnosis?

Pancreatitis, AAA, cholecystitis, bowel obstruction/perforation, diabetic ketoacidosis, perforated enteric ulcer.

How would you initially manage this patient?

The patient should be stabilised following an ABCDE approach with oxygen supplementation, IV access with two large-bore cannulas and fluid resuscitation. Life threatening haemodynamic compromise requires identification and correction. The patient may require catheterisation to monitor fluid balance and appropriate analgesia should be administered to ensure the patient is comfortable.

History taking, clinical examination and basic investigations including imaging will all help identify the underlying condition.

What investigations would you order?

Bloods including FBC, U&E, LFTs, serum amylase, lipase and an ABG.
Erect CXR: Pneumoperitoneum is not present.
AXR: Loss of psoas shadow indicates retroperitoneal fluid.
USS: Gallstones, pancreatic fluid. No AAA.
CT Abdomen: Pancreatic inflammation and fluid.

The patient's amlylase comes back as 985Iu/mL.

A CT scan has been ordered

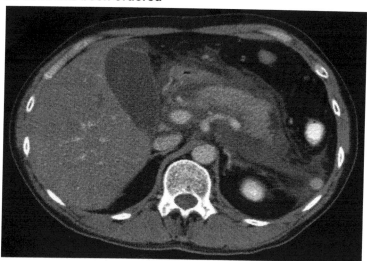

APPLIED SCIENCES

What does the CT scan show?

This is an axial cut CT scan at the level of the pancreas, liver and gallbladder. There is fluid surrounding the pancreas and the outline of the pancreas is only just visible suggesting acute inflammation rather than progression to necrosis.

What are the causes of acute pancreatitis?

Remembered by the mnemonic: **I GET SMASHED**

I - Idiopathic
G - Gallstones (60%)
E - Ethanol (30%)
T - Trauma
S - Steroids
M - Mumps
A - Autoimmune - e.g. SLE
S - Scorpion bites (rare!)
H - Hypercalcaemia, hypothermia, hyperlipidaemia
E - ERCP
D - Drugs - e.g. NSAIDs, thiazides, azathioprine, isoniazid

90% of acute pancreatitis cases are caused by alcohol, gallstones, ERCP or are idiopathic.

What is the likely cause in this case and why is it important?

Given the history of a heavy drinking session alcohol seems the most likely cause. Diagnosis of the underlying cause affects the ultimate management of the patient. Additionally in the case of alcohol care must be taken to appropriately treat the patient for alcohol withdrawal using the local hospital protocol. This is usually chlordiazepoxide and a Vitamin B12 reducing regime. An ultrasound scan is useful in all patients to ensure there is not concurrent gallstone disease. However it is important to remember that this can be an incidental finding.

What scoring systems do you know to classify severity of acute pancreatitis?

APACHE II, Ranson, BISAP and Glasgow. The modified Glasgow (Imrie) score is the most widely used to assess prognostic severity.

What would your long-term management be?

Management is largely supportive and patients often require admission to ITU for careful fluid resuscitation.
Other supportive measures include nasogastric suction to prevent abdominal distention and vomiting. Continuous oxygen may be required. Enteral nutrition must be commenced, there appears to be no clear benefit of nasojejunal over nasogastric feeding, parenteral feeding should only be utilised if enteral feeding fails to meet demands.

What are some of the complications of acute pancreatitis?

Pancreatic pseudocyst, pancreatic necrosis, chronic pancreatitis, ARDS, SIRS, death.

What is believed to be the role of calcium in the pathogenesis pancreatitis?

Regardless of initial insult it is believed that the final common pathway is a marked increase in intracellular calcium, which causes activation of intracellular proteases. Proteases digest the walls of blood vessels causing blood extravasation and amylase is released into the blood. Released lipases cause fat necrosis within the abdomen and subcutaneous tissue. The released fatty acids can bind to calcium and cause hypocalcaemia. Concomitant destruction of adjacent islet cells can produce hyperglycaemia and thus cause diabetes. Cullens and Grey-Turners sign are secondary to retroperitoneal or intra-abdominal bleeding as a result of leaked pancreatic enzymes.

The patient is admitted to ITU and becomes breathless. A CXR is arranged:

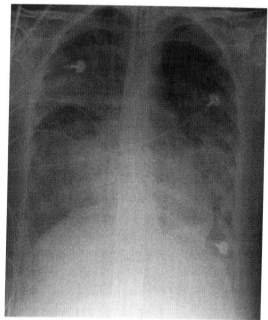

Describe the radiograph

The erect CXR demonstrates diffuse, patchy pulmonary infiltrates throughout both lung fields. There is a correctly sited Endotracheal tube, left subclavian line, right internal jugular line, nasogastric tube and ECG lines. There is also an artefact on the left proximal humerus, this could possibly be an intra-osseous needle.

What is the likely diagnosis?

Given the history of pancreatitis acute respiratory distress syndrome(ARDS) is the likely diagnosis.

What is the definition of ARDS?

ARDS is a severe form of acute lung injury (ALI) secondary to diffuse alveolar injury. ARDS is defined by the Berlin definition as:
Lung injury of acute onset, within 1 week of an apparent clinical insult and with progression of respiratory symptoms
Bilateral opacities on chest imaging not explained by other lung pathology

APPLIED SCIENCES

Respiratory failure not explained by heart failure or volume overload (non-cardiogenic, normal wedge pressure)

Decreased arterial PaO2/FiO2 ratio

What is the pathophysiology behind ARDS?

There is an inflammatory component to ARDS, caused by neutrophils and macrophages. They release mediators that activate the complement and coagulation cascades. The result is an increase in endothelial permeability and pulmonary oedema. This causes hypoxaemia.

How would you manage the patient now?

Treatment of the underlying cause is paramount. The respiratory system must concurrently be supported and this is often via mechanical ventilation in the Intensive Care Unit. Ventilation is usually delivered through oro-tracheal intubation, or in some units by tracheostomy if prolonged ventilation is deemed likely. Ventilation can be challenging however lung protective ventilation is attempted. Other strategies include application of PEEP, prone ventilation and high frequency oscilation. Some may use extra-corporeal membrane oxygenation (ECMO). The optimum strategy is currently debated. Alongside the aforementioned good ITU care such as nutrition, optimal fluid administration, organ support and early detection and treatment of secondary problems such as ventilator associated pneumonia is key.

SUMMARY

Glasgow Imrie classification of pancreatitis:

PaO2	<8kPa
Age	>55 years
Neutrophils	>15x109/L
Calcium	<2mmol/L
Renal function	Urea >16mmol/L
Enzymes	LDH >600iU/L or AST >200iU/L
Albumin	<32g/L
Sugar	>10mmol/L

TOP TIPS

➕ The Glasgow Imrie classification can be recalled by the mnemonic PANCREAS

➕ ARDS needs management on ITU and is a life-threatening condition not to be missed

1.4 Pulmonary Embolus

Scenario

You are called to review a 67 year old man on the elective orthopaedic ward 5 days following a right total hip replacement. He is complaining of shortness of breath and his saturations are 92% on room air. His past medical history includes hypertension and type 2 diabetes controlled with oral hypoglycaemics. His wound has been requiring daily dressing changes due to oozing and therefore he has not had low molecular weight heparin (LMWH) for the last two days.

What would be your initial management of this patient?

Initial management would consist of assessing the patient using the model of airway, breathing, circulation and treating any abnormality as it is identified. The first part of management would be to apply high flow oxygen via a non-rebreathe mask. His notes should also be reviewed at the bedside and basic bedside tests such as an ECG performed.

What are your differential diagnoses?

This patient may have a pulmonary embolism, atelectasis, pneumonia or pulmonary oedema. Given he has not received anticoagulation a pulmonary embolism should be high on the list of differentials.

Observations show RR 21/min, Saturations 96% on 15L O2, HR 112/min, BP 103/76. Temperature 37.8

He has good air entry bilaterally with no added sounds. Heart sounds are normal, and his pulse is regular. His right leg is swollen with pitting oedema to the level of above the knee.

What management would you initiate?

He should remain on high flow oxygen to maintain saturations of greater than 94% as long as there is no history of chronic lung disease which may have resulted in a reliance on hypoxic drive. IV fluids should be started, initially with a 250-500ml bolus of Hartmann's solution. Observations should be rechecked after this fluid bolus to check response. Ongoing monitoring of fluid status will be required, sometimes this may require urethral catheterisation however in the elderly this can in itself result in delirium and other further complications.

What investigations would you request?

A full set of blood tests including FBC, U&E, CRP and clotting studies along with an ABG should be taken. He requires an ECG and CXR and a CTPA if the CXR does not show another cause for the symptoms. A D-Dimer is not indicated as it will be raised secondary to surgery.
If he were pyrexic blood cultures would be indicated.

The ABG on 15L shows pH 7.52, PaO2 9.7kPa, PaCO2 3.1kPa, HCO3 21, BE 4.1

How would you interpret this ABG?

This patient has a Type 1 Respiratory Failure, as shown by the low PaO2. You would expect this to be much higher given the amount of oxygen being given. There is also a respiratory alkalosis demonstrated by the raised pH and low PaCO2. There is partial metabolic compensation as the HCO3 is marginally low.

How would this ABG affect your diagnosis and management?

This confirms that the patient is hypoxic. Given that they have a respiratory alkalosis it makes it more likely that the cause is a PE. A CTPA would be the next appropriate investigation.

What signs might an ECG demonstarte in a patient with a PE?

This ECG might show sinus tachycardia. The classical picture of S1Q3T3 is seen in pulmonary embolism. There is a Q wave in III, prominent S wave in I and T wave inversion in III, V1 and V2.

How would you approach looking at an ECG?

You need a systematic method for analysing ECGs. Check for sinus rhythm by looking for P, QRS and T waves all appearing. Decide whether the rhythm is regular or irregular. Calculate the rate by dividing 300 by the number of big squares between each QRS complex. Calculate the axis of the ECG. Then look in turn at PR interval for conduction defects, QRS duration for bundle branch block and any changes in ST segment or T wave morphology. Finally you need to compare to any previous available ECGs.

You go on to request the CTPA for the patient which confirms a right sided PE

How would this alter your management?

With a confirmed PE resuscitation with IV fluid is still required, but anticoagulation also needs to be started. In post-operative patients it may be wise to inform the operating surgeon of the need for anticoagulation. In the first instance low molecular weight heparin is started at a treatment dose, with conversion to either Warfarin or a novel oral anticoagulant according to local policy.

What are the factors that contribute to thrombosis?

Virchow's triad explains the three factors that contribute to thrombosis formation; they are hypercoagulability, stasis and endothelial injury.

What is the pathophysiology behind the hypoxia associated with PE?

In a PE there is V/Q mismatch caused by impaired perfusion of the affected segment. This causes an increase in perfusion of the normal parts of the lung; however there is no increase in ventilation to these overperfused areas. Segments can become infarcted due to obstruction of the arterial system, and is more common in patients with pre-existing cardio-respiratory disease. When this does occur it leads to pleuritic chest pain and haemoptysis. Pulmonary hypertension is associated with massive PE and is secondary to increased right ventricular afterload. Pulmonary artery systolic pressure increases in order

APPLIED SCIENCES

to maintain cardiac output.

What is the mechanism of action of Warfarin?

It inhibits Vitamin K reductase therefore prevents the production of Vitamin K dependent clotting factors II, VII, IX and X.

How long would the patient require Warfarin?

3 months as there is a clear temporary risk factor, and then the need should be reassessed.

If a patient presents to the pre-assessment clinic taking Warfarin how would you manage them around the time of their operation?

Management depends on the indication for their Warfarin treatment. The risk of them developing thrombosis whilst off anticoagulation should be calculated. They should stop the Warfarin 5 days prior to the surgery, and instead receive low molecular weight Heparin pre-operatively and post-operatively whilst the Warfarin is re-loaded. If the patient has a metallic heart valve they may require unfractionated Heparin instead.

If a patient is on Warfarin when they are admitted requiring emergency surgery how would this be treated?

The INR should be checked. Ideally it should be below 1.5 to allow surgery to go ahead. If there is enough time to reverse the INR with Vitamin K this can be given either orally or intravenously usually at a dose of between 1 and 5mg. In life threatening bleeding prothrombin complex concentrate can be given.

What alternatives to Warfarin are there and what are the considerations of these drugs?

Novel oral anticoagulants such as Rivaroxaban and Dabigatran are recent options. There is no way of reversing these, and clearance is via the renal system. Therefore the patient's renal function should be considered when it comes to thinking about excretion of these drugs. Local policies will give guidance on the length of time that should be left following the last dose before operating.

APPLIED SCIENCES

SUMMARY

Pulmonary embolism and deep vein thrombosis (DVT) are manifestations of venous thromboembolism. The majority of pulmonary emboli arise from the legs in particular the proximal veins (i.e. popliteal and above).

Dislodged thrombi pass through the right side of the heart and become trapped in the pulmonary vasculature. Physical obstruction leads to increased pulmonary vascular resistance and right ventricular (RV) afterload. Compensatory mechanisms result in right ventricular dilatation and a reduction in RV cardiac output. As a result there is a reduction in left ventricular (LV) preload and an overall drop in cardiac output, which is manifested as hypotension and shock.

APPLIED SCIENCES

TOP TIPS

➕ Pleuritic pain is particularly associated with distal small emboli. Large central emboli typically result in respiratory distress and cardiovascular collapse.

➕ Inferior vena cava filters *(IVC)* block emboli from reaching the lungs. They can be considered in patients with DVT who cannot be given anticoagulants.

➕ Thrombophilia screen should be performed in patients with unprovoked PE. However this should be done after anti-coagulation is stopped as it is impossible to interpret the results in the presence of anticoagulation.

➕ If warfarin is given without heparin it may paradoxically increase hypercoagulability.

Further Reading:
1. BTS guidelines. (2003). British Thoracic Society guidelines for the management of suspected pulmonary embolism
2. NICE. Anticoagulation - Oral. Clinical Knowledge Summaries: NICE; 2015.

1.5 | Crush Injury

Scenario

A 50 year old man is brought into the emergency department following a road traffic accident. He was a pedestrian hit by a car and trapped beneath the wheels for approximately 45 minutes whilst waiting to be freed. He has been assessed using the ATLS algorithm and the only injuries noted are a swollen right calf.

What investigations would you request?

Blood tests including a FBC, U&E's and CK are required. Venous blood gas in ED would be useful. A group and save should be taken in preparation for potential surgery. An initial x ray of the leg can rule out fractures.

The blood results are shown below:

Hb 146 g/L   Na 131 mmol/L   CK 3800 U/L
WCC 10.8 x109/L   K 5.0 mmol/L
Plt 271 x109/L   Ur 9.3 mmol/L
Cr 198 mmol/L

What do these blood results show and what is the likely diagnosis?

There is a raised CK, which is diagnostic of rhabdomyolysis. The patient also has a raised urea and creatinine which indicates renal impairment. Potassium is also marginally raised in keeping with rhabdomyolysis. Rhabdomyolysis in this case is most likely secondary to the crush injury.

What is rhabdomyolysis?

Rhabdomyolysis is a syndrome where muscle necrosis leads to the release of intracellular contents into the systemic circulation. Notably creatine kinase, muscle enzymes, myoglobin and potassium. It is associated with muscle pain, weakness, dark coloured urine and raised serum creatine kinase levels.

What are the common causes of rhabdomyolysis?

Prolonged lie, crush injury, reperfusion syndrome, burns, excessive exercise and hyper/hypothermia. Drugs such as statins can also result in rhabdomyolysis.

What are the complications of rhabdomyolysis?

It can lead to electrolyte imbalances (hyperkalaemia), acute kidney injury and compartment syndrome.

How does rhabdomyolysis cause acute kidney injury?

Myoglobin is released from damaged muscle cells and causes damage to the renal tubules as it accumulates. Further to this extracellular fluid is redistributed into the muscle resulting in hypovolaemia.

APPLIED SCIENCES

How can acute kidney injury be prevented in patients with a crush injury?

The treatment of rhabdomyolysis is primarily to prevent renal failure with aggressive fluid administration being the primary treatment modality, a urine output of 200-300ml/hour is aimed for. However this must be weighed up against risk such as in CCF patients. Alkalinisation of the urine and diuretic therapy are also potential treatment options, however evidence for this is mixed. If patients don't respond to fluid administration haemodialysis is indicated.

On rechecking the renal function the potassium has increased to 7.2

What ECG changes are associated with hyperkalaemia?

It is associated with small P waves, wide QRS complexes and tall tented T waves. In some cases this can progress to VF.

How would you treat hyperkalaemia of this level?

10mL of 10% calcium gluconate is used to stabilise cardiac muscle. IV Insulin and Dextrose promotes cellular uptake of potassium as does nebulised Salbutamol. Calcium resonium works on a longer term basis to promote excretion of potassium.

In the unstable patient or those who fail to respond to medical treatment haemodialysis/haemofiltration should be considered.

What is compartment syndrome?

An increase in the pressure within an osseofascial compartment.

What is the pathophysiology of compartment syndrome?

There is an increase in the pressure within a compartment to greater than the venous pressure. This obstructs the venous return and therefore increases the pressure further as blood is unable to leave. Eventually this becomes greater than the arterial pressure preventing oxygen delivery to the muscles. Muscle necrosis occurs.

What are the commonest causes of compartment syndrome?

It is commonly associated with diaphyseal fractures, especially of the tibia. It can also be caused by coagulopathies causing haematoma, rhabdomyolysis, tight bandaging and arterial injury. Remember that compartment syndrome can still occur in the presence of an open fracture.

How would you demonstrate compartment syndrome in the leg?

Clinically the patient would be in a lot of pain, often out of proportion to the injury sustained. Pain increases on passive stretch of the affected compartment. Findings of reduced peripheral pulses and altered sensation are late signs and indicate that the diagnosis has been delayed.

How could you diagnose compartment syndrome in a patient on ITU?

If clinical signs can't be elicited because the patient is unconscious compartment pressure monitoring can be used. This involves measuring the pressure within each compartment of the affected limb. If the pressure is within 30mmHg of the diastolic blood pressure it is compartment syndrome.

How should compartment syndrome be managed?

Compartment syndrome is an emergency, requiring urgent surgical decompression of the compartments. In the leg there are four compartments; all can be decompressed through two incisions. One is antero-lateral to release the anterior and lateral compartments. The second is postero-medial to decompress the superficial and deep posterior compartments. Muscle belly bulging through the wound is diagnostic of compartment syndrome. Any non-viable muscle should be debrided. The wounds should be left open initially, with either an attempt at closure in a planned second stage or plastic surgery input to graft the area.

SUMMARY

Rhabdomyolysis is a potentially life-threatening syndrome that can develop from a variety of causes; the classic findings of muscular aches, weakness and tea-coloured urine are non-specific and may not always be present. the diagnosis therefore rests upon the presence of a high level of suspicion of any abnormal laboratory values in the mind of the treating physician. An elevated plasma creatine kinase (CK) level is the most sensitive laboratory finding pertaining to muscle injury; whereas hyperkalaemia, acute renal failure and compartment syndrome represent the major life-threatening complications. The management of the condition includes prompt and aggressive fluid resuscitation, elimination of the causative agents and treatment and prevention of any complications that may ensue.

Compartment syndrome is an orthopaedic emergency. Compartment syndrome is a process where the pressure within a myofascial compartment exceeds the perfusion pressure of that compartment. This can be caused by factors external to the compartment, such as a tight cast or skin contractures following a burn, or by internal factors such as swelling following a fracture or blunt injury.

The presenting feature is pain, pain and more pain. The pain will be out of proportion to the injury sustained. Review the drug card to see how much pain relief has been given – it is usually lots. The pain is usually within the muscle compartment rather than at the fracture site and is exacerbated on passive stretch of the muscle. Other features are late and herald that the compartment syndrome has been missed. A lack of pulses suggests a vascular injury and need to be documented and an opinion from a vascular surgeon obtained. Pale palor and paraesthesia indicate tissue ischaemia and the need to get a good lawyer. If you suspect compartment syndrome, take a quick history and make the patient nil by mouth in anticipation of surgery. Cut any cast, dressing or splint down to skin – do not leave any wool or padding as this alone can cause significant pressure. Keep the limb at the level of the heart, high elevation will reduce the perfusion pressure while dangling the limb low will increase swelling. Give a dose of morphine and call the registrar. If the pain does not resolve with these conservative measures then the patient will need to go to theatre for a fasciotomy.

It is useful to know how to measure compartment pressures, which can be found in the skill station. Compartment pressures are useful when the patient is unconscious following major injury or cannot give a pain response. Compartment syndrome is present if the pressure is more than 30mmHg, or the difference in pressure (diastolic blood pressure – compartment pressure) is less than 30mmHg.

APPLIED SCIENCES

TOP TIPS

✚ Compartment syndrome is a clinical diagnosis but pressure monitors may be of help if there is any uncertainty or the patient is unconscious.

✚ Rhabdomyolysis is a potentially life-threatening condition and should be considered in anyone who has been lying unconscious for any period of time or who has suffered a crush mechanism of injury.

Further Reading:
1. BMJ. Rhabdomyolysis: Management. BMJ Best Practice
2. Shuler M, Roskosky M, Freedman B. Compartment Syndromes. In: Bruce B, ed. Skeletal Trauma: Saunder; 2015:437-463.

1.6 Transurethral Resection of Prostate

Scenario

A 64 year old man underwent a TURP for BPH earlier today. You are called to see him on the ward due to confusion and nausea. He is usually fit with no co-morbidities and no regular medications. A set of observations is performed: RR 15, Saturations 98% on air, HR 94/min, BP 165/97.

What is a TURP?

A TURP is a trans-urethral resection of the prostate. This uses large volumes of fluid to irrigate the urethra and electrocautery to resect the prostate.

What is BPH?

Benign prostatic hyperplasia.

What is the cellular pathology behind hyperplasia?

In hyperplasia there is an increase in the number of cells but they remain of a normal size. This is compared to hypertrophy in which the size of the cell increases but the number remains stable.

What are your differential diagnoses of this patient's symptoms?

This patient may have TURP syndrome. Differentials may include complications related to a general anaesthesia (such as post operative delirium, CVA, ACS) or side effects secondary to his analgesia.

What is TURP syndrome?

TURP syndrome is a collection of symptoms including nausea, confusion, disorientation, seizures, visual disturbances (especially if glycine irrigant) and signs of fluid overload (including pulmonary oedema). It is caused by intravenous absorption of nonconductive (electrolyte-free) irrigation fluid during the procedure resulting in a hyponatraemia. It occurs in between 1 and 8% of TURP cases.

What fluids are used for irrigation in a TURP?

Non-electrolyte/non-conductive solutions such as Glycine 1.5% are used during the procedure in order to allow monopolar electrocautery devices to be used.

What is the pathogenesis of TURP syndrome?

The symptoms are caused by a dilutional hyponatraemia following absorption of irrigation fluid. The volume that is absorbed is directly correlated to the degree of hyponatraemia. The rate of absorption also affects hyponatraemia; the solution is absorbed more quickly if there is damage to blood vessels and therefore increased intravasation of the solution. Most irrigation fluids are nearly isotonic, however there are hypotonic solutions which also cause a dilutionaly hyponatraemia.

How might you prevent TURP syndrome?

APPLIED SCIENCES

There are certain measures one can put in place in order to minimise the risk of developing TURP syndrome. These consist of the following:
• Limit the duration (time) of irrigation and monitor the fluid absorbtion (amount instilled – amount removed). If a pre-determined time or value is reached the procedure should be stopped.
• Using an electrolyte containing isotonic solution. This limits one to a diagnostic procedure or a therapy using a bipolar diathermy .
• Limit the intravesical pressure.

How would you manage this patient?

The patient should be assessed using the ABCDE approach. An urgent set of bloods to check electrolytes and serum osmolality should be sent. Management is mainly supportive with fluid restriction, and consists of adequate monitoring often in a high dependency unit. If the diagnosis is made intra-operatively the surgery must be stopped.

IV fluids should be stopped, oxygen applied and the patient assessed for the need of additional respiratory support. Furosemide can be used if acute pulmonary oedema complicates the condition, hypertonic saline can be used if sodium is severely low. Sodium must be corrected slowly to prevent central pontine myelinolysis.

How would you assess the patient for confusion?

The AMTS (Abbreviated Mental Test Score) is a set of 10 standard questions used to record/quantify the level of confusion. It is easily replicated and has a high sensitivity for diagnosing memory impairment.

Where is the majority of sodium found in the body?

It is an extracellular ion with the majority being found extracellulary.

How would you classify hypoosmolar hyponatraemia?

Hyponatraemia can be classified depending on fluid status into three categories;
• Hypervolaemic
• Euvolaemic
• Hypovolaemic

What causes hypervolaemic hypoosmolar hyponatraemia?

TURP syndrome would fit into this category. Other causes include cardiac failure, nephrotic syndrome and liver cirrhosis.

What is SIADH?

SIADH stands for Syndrome of Inappropriate Anti-Diuretic Hormone (ADH) secretion and can be associated with many disorders. An excess of ADH is present which results in an increased retention of water by the collecting ducts of the kidney. There is loss of the negative feedback system which would usually reduce the amount of ADH secreted as the plasma osmolality decreases and thus there is a failure to supress continued ADH release. This results in a euvolaemic hyponatraemia.

What causes a hypovolaemic hypoosmolar hyponatraemia?

Examples include inappropriate diuretic use, Addison's disease, diarrhoea and vomiting.

SUMMARY

Transurethral resection of the prostate (TURP) is a surgery used to treat urinary problems due to an enlarged prostate.

A combined visual and surgical instrument (resectoscope) is inserted through the tip of the penis and into the urethra. It is used to 'trim' away excess prostate tissue that is compressing the lumen.

TURP is generally considered an option for men with moderate to severe urinary problems that haven't responded to medication. Traditionally, TURP has been considered the most effective treatment for an enlarged prostate.

Transurethral Resection of the Prostate (TURP) Syndrome is a rare but potentially life-threatening complication of a transurethral resection of the prostate procedure. It occurs as a consequence of the absorption into the prostatic venous sinuses of the fluids used to irrigate the bladder during the operation.

The symptoms are caused by a dilutional hyponatraemia following absorption of irrigation fluid. The volume that is absorbed is directly correlated to the degree of hyponatraemia. The rate of absorption also affects hyponatraemia; the solution is absorbed more quickly if there is damage to blood vessels and therefore increased intravasation of the solution. Most irrigation fluids are nearly isotonic, however there are hypotonic solutions which also cause a dilutionaly hyponatraemia.

TOP TIPS

➕ TURP is a common procedure and one should be confident with its indications, be able to describe the procedures and be aware of some potential complications.

➕ Hyponatraemia is often a confusing area however it is important to be able to classify each type and understand broad principles and simple management strategies.

APPLIED SCIENCES

1.7 Gastric Outlet Obstruction

Scenario

A 56 year old with a history of peptic ulceration presents with a 24 hour history of persistent vomiting. His arterial blood gas results are shown below:

PaO2	12.4 kPa	(>10 kPa on air)
pH	7.59	(7.35 – 7.45)
PaCO2	6.1 kPa	(4.5 – 6.0 kPa)
HCO3–	50.1 mmol/ L	(22 – 26 mmol/ L)
BE -	25 mmol/ L	(+/- 2 mmol/ L)
K+	2.9 mmol/ L	(3.5 – 5 mmol/ L)
Na+	136 mmol/ L	(135 – 145 mmol/ L)
Cl-	77 mmol/ L	(95 – 105 mmol/ L)

What is your differential diagnosis?

This patient's history and blood gas results are suggestive of gastric outlet obstruction. Key causes of gastric outlet obstruction are:

Benign	Malignant
• Peptic ulcer disease o Secondary to inlfamation/oedema or scarring • Infections: Tuberculosis and infiltrative diseases such as amyloidosis. • Congenital pyloric stenosis • Pancreatic pseudocyst • Polyp • Bouveret's syndrome (obstruction due to a gallstone) (rare) • Pyloric mucosal diaphragm (rare)	• Adenocarcinoma of the stomach • Lymphoma • Pancreatic carcinoma • Gastrointestinal stromal tumours

How would you initially manage this patient?

The patient should be stabilised following an ABCDE approach with identification and correction of life-threatening haemodynamic parameters. They require intravenous access with two large-bore cannulas and fluid resuscitation. Catheterisation should be considered to monitor fluid balance and urine output.

Appropriate antiemetics should be administered to minimise further vomiting. An ECG should also be performed in view of the hypokalaemia and this should be corrected with intravenous potassium with normal saline. A wide bore naso-gastric tube should be passed.

Identification of the underlying condition and cause should then follow by taking a history and examining the patient. Emergent treatment of the underlying cause and supportive resuscitation and fluid balance will be the mainstay of ongoing treatment.

What do this patients initial blood tests show?

There is a severe metabolic alkalosis with attempted respiratory compensation. The sodium is low/normal and there is loss of both potassium and chloride ions. This can be described as a hypochloremic-hypokalemic metabolic alkalosis.

Explain how gastric outlet obstruction causes the above results?

• Gastric outflow obstruction causes a progressive metabolic alkalosis that is perpetuated by the normal compensatory mechanisms.

• Gastric losses: Gastric secretions are rich in hydrogen and chloride ions. To facilitate the secretion of hydrogen and chloride ions bicarbonate is formed within the parietal cell. The bicarbonate is moved into the interstitum (and ultimately the plasma) via a chloride/bicarbonate antiporter. As gastric secretions are lost secretion must continue to replace that which is lost, which means bicarbonate production continues. This contributes to an alkalosis as hydrogen is lost and bicarbonate produced and moved into the interstitium.

• Reduced duodenal acid load: there is a reduction of pancreatic exocrine secretions due to the reduced acid load at the duodenum. This leads to retention of bicarbonate-rich pancreatic secretion.

• Volume depletion and renal response: Initially the increased bicarbonate is excreted in the urine. However as volume depletion arises aldosterone is released. This increases sodium reabsorbtion and therefore bicarbonate reabsorbtion along with hydrogen and potassium loss.

Remember that as in all states of volume depleteion AKI can occur.

The nurse sends off a urine sample which shows an aciduria. Why is this?

Due to aldosterone released secondary to volume depletion, bicarbonate is reabsorbed and hydrogen lost into the urine resulting in the paradoxical finding of aciduria.

What cells are found within the stomach and what do they secrete?

• Parietal cells: secretion of hydrochloric acid and intrinsic factor.
• Chief cells: secretion of pepsinogen (the precursor of pepsin) and gastric lipase
• Mucous cells: secrete mucus
• G-cells: secrete the hormone gastrin

What is the average daily volume of gastric secretion?

The average volume of daily gastric secretion is 1-1.5L.

What is the role of hydrochloric acid when secreted?

• Hydrochloric acid has some proteolytic activity
• Results in a pH of approximately 2 which provides the ideal environment for the gastric enzyme pepsin
• Has antibacterial properties and prevents colonisation

Outline how hydrochloric acid is secreted from parietal cells and by what means this is regulated.

Carbon dioxide diffuses into the cell and via cytoplasmic carbonic anhydrase with water froms carbonic acid, this then dissociates into bicarbonate and hydrogen. Bicarbonate is then lost from the cell into the interstitium via a basolateral bicarbonate/chloride antiporter, thus chloride ions move into the cell. The hydrogen is actively transported via a hydrogen/ potassium ATPase into the gastric lumen. The potassium transported into the cell during this exchange then passes back into the gastric lumen via apical potassium channels. Chloride ions move out of the cell into the gastric lumen via apical chloride channels

Hydrochloric acid secretion is stimulated by:
- Acetylcholine from parasympathetic vagal neurones that innervate the parietal cells directly
- Gastrin produced by pyloric G-cells
- Histamine produced by enterochromaffin-like cells. This stimulates the parietal cells directly and also potentiates parietal cell stimulation by gastrin and neuronal stimulation

Hydrochloric acid secretion is inhibited by:
- Somatostatin release from D-cells in response to a pH
- Secretin produced by the duodenum
- Cholecystokinin

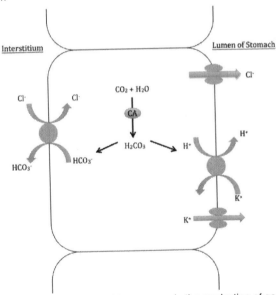

Figure 17.1: A pictoral representation of key process in the production of gastric acid at the parietal cellular level. Produced by Mr C Handford.

Describe the process and phases of gastric acid secretion

Cephalic phase
Initiated by the thought, smell, sight and taste of food. Leads to vagal activation that stimulates hydrochloric acid and gastrin secretion.

Gastric phase
Stretch and chemoreceptors are activated by the presence of food in the stomach par-

ticularly protein rich food. There is again an increase in the level of gastric secretions and gastrin. In this phase the tone of the lower oesophageal sphincter increases to prevent reflux and peristalsis increases.

Intestinal phase

Only accounts for 10% of gastric acid production. Initially the chyme, especially the amino acids, in the duodenum stimulates acid production by a poorly understood pathway not mediated by serum gastrin but possibly by another hormone called entero-oxyntin. Following this a comination of gastric inhibitory protein (GIP), secretin and cholecystokinin (CCK) inhibit gastric acid secretion, mobilitiy and emptying.

What are the functions of gastrin?

- Stimulates gastric acid secretion
- Stimulates growth of gastic mucosa
- Stimulates gastric motility
- Stimulates exocrine pancreatic secretions

What is the storage capacity of the stomach?

The stomach can store approximately 1-2L.

Describe the autonomic nervous supply to the stomach

- Sympathetic: From the coeliac plexus, reduces gastric motility
- Parasympathetic: From the vagus nerve causing increased motility

Which key hormones contribute to emptying of the stomach?

- Promote gastric emptying
     o Gastrin

- Inhibit gastric empytying
     o Cholecystokinin
     o Gastric inhibitory protein

Describe the process of vomiting

- Highly coordinated reflex process.
- This process is coordinated by the vomiting centre of the medulla, and influences directly by afferent innervaton and indirectly via the chemoreceptor trigger zone.
- Split into 2 phases.
- Pre-ejection phase:
     o Nausae experienced.
     o Increased sympathetic activity therefore become tachycaridic, sweaty.
     o Parasympathetic activity means the salivation increases, the oesophageal sphincters relax and there is a retrograde conctraction.
- Ejection phase
     o Mid inspiration a breath is held
     o The hyoid and larynx are raised to open the crico-oesophageal sphincter
     o The glottis closes
     o Contraction of the diaphragm and abdominal musculature raises the pressure in the stomach
     o The diaphragmatic hiatus relaxes and oesophageal sphincters open which force the contents into the oesophagus and out of the body. Alongside this as the gastric contents enters the oesophagus there is retrograde contraction of the striated muscle of the oesophagus

APPLIED SCIENCES

SUMMARY

Gastric outlet obstruction can cause severe and persistent vomiting resulting in a hypochloraemic hypokalaemic metabolic alkalosis. Immediate management should focus on fluid resuscitation and correction of the patients' electrolytes.

There are three phases to gastric acid secretion: the cephalic phase, gastric phase and the intestinal phase.

Individuals with gastric outlet obstruction will often have recurrent vomiting of food that has accumulated in the stomach, but which cannot pass into the small intestine due to the obstruction. The stomach often dilates to accommodate food intake and secretions.

Causes of gastric outlet obstruction include both benign causes (such as peptic ulcer disease affecting the area around the pylorus), as well as malignant causes, such as gastric cancer.

Treatment of the condition depends upon the underlying cause; it can involve antibiotic treatment when Helicobacter pylori is related to an ulcer, endoscopic therapies (such as dilation of the obstruction with balloons or the placement of self expandable metallic stents), other medical therapies, or surgery to resolve the obstruction.

APPLIED SCIENCES

TOP TIPS

➕ Abdominal imaging should be considered in gastric outlet obstruction to exclude an underlying malignancy and endoscopy is useful to help vislaise the outlet and provide the ability to take tissue samples or relieve the obstruction.

➕ Early discussion with intensive care may be required if patients with gastric outlet obstruction have severe electrolyte derangement or haemodynamic instability.

➕ Ensure that patients have not developed an Acute Kidney Injury due to significant dehydration.

1.8 Hypercalcaemia

Scenario

A 40 year old male presents with a 12 hour history of intermittent right loin pain radiating to the groin. On examination he has a heart rate of 110bpm and he has right renal angle tenderness.

What is your differential diagnosis?

- Renal colic
- Pyelonephritis
- Papillary necrosis
- Renal tumour
- Renal infarction
- AAA
- Retroperitoneal fibrosis

How would you initially manage this patient?

The patient should be stabilised following an ABCDE approach with identification and correction of life-threatening findings. They require IV access with two large-bore cannulas with fluid resuscitation.

The patients' fluid balance should be monitored and appropriate analgesia and antiemetics administered.

Identification of the underlying cause should be sought by taking a history and thouroughly examining the patient.

What investigations would you order/consider?

- Bloods: FBC, U&E, LFTs, CRP, serum amylase, bone profile, VBG. If pyrexic cultures would be needed.
- Urine dipstick (with pregnancy test if female)
- Imaging: Ideally CT KUB however plain film radiograph is an alternative. Bedside USS of the aorta is quick and easy to carry out in the patients bay if a AAA is suspected.

Following administration of analgesia he is afebrile with normal observations. His urine dip is only positive for microscopic haematuria and his initial blood test results are shown below:

Urea	6.2	(2.5 – 6.7 mmol/ L)
Creatinine	95	(70 – 130 µmol/ L)
White cell count	8.2	(4 -11 x 109/ L)
C-reactive protein	8	(0-10)

A plain film KUB radiograph is performed and there is no abnormality detectable.

APPLIED SCIENCES

What percentage of renal calculi are radio-opaque?

Approximately 90% of renal calculi are radio-opaque.

Given the clinical history and initial investigations the patient undergoes a CT KUB. It shows a right sided 6mm stone at the vesico-ureteric junction with no evidence of hydronephrosis.

What are the most common sites where renal calculi can cause obstruction?

There are 3 common sites where renal calculi can cause obstruction. They are:
• Pelvic-ureteric junction
• Site where the ureter crosses the pelvic brim
• Vesico-ureteric junction

How should this patient be managed?

The patient should be given appropriate analgesia. In patients with renal colic NSAIDs are thought to be particularly effective analgesia. NSAIDs prevent afferent arteriolar vasodilatation (by inhibiting prostaglandin synthesis) reducing diuresis and thus reducing distal pressures in the urinary tract and minimising stimulation of stretch receptors. They also minimise oedema and inflammation. All of these factors combined minimse ureteric activity and help reduce pain. Alongside these NSAIDs may also relax the ureteric smooth muscle. The most commonly used NSAID in renal colic is PR diclofenac. Other analgesics including parenteral opiates may be required. Anti-emetics should also be considered.

This patient has a renal calculi that is less than 10mm which is likely to pass spontaneously. He has normal renal function with no hydronpehrosis. Additionally there is no evidence to suggest that this ureteric obstruction has led to pyelonephritis. Once his pain is controlled he can therefore be managed conservatively. This may include the use of medical expulsive therapy by the use of an alpha-blocker e.g. tamsulosin to facilitate spontaneous stone passage.

The patient should be followed up in the urology clinic 2-3 weeks after discharge. He should be advised to collect the stone if possible so that it can be sent for analysis and to return if the pain becomes uncontrollable or he becomes unwell.

Two weeks later he returns to clinic. His symptoms have improved. Repeat blood tests show the following.

Albumin	45 g/ L	(35- 50 g/ L)
Calcium	2.85 mmol/ L	(2.12 – 2.65 mmol/ L)

What is this patients' corrected calcium level?

40% of serum calcium is albumin bound. Variations in albumin concentration and therefore, total plasma calcium may not accurately reflect the concentration of ionized calcium. The corrected calcium level allows for the change in total calcium due to the change in albumin bound calcium. The following equation can be used to calculate corrected calcium levels:

Corrected calcium(mmol/L) = measured total Calcium(mmol/L) + 0.02 (40 - serum albumin[g/L])

40 represents the average albumin level in g/L

This patient's corrected calcium is therefore 2.75 mmol/ L

What are the causes of hypercalcaemia?

• Hyperparathyroidism (primary and tertiary)
• Malignancy (direct metastases to bone causing lysis or hypercalcaemia due to circulating parathyroid hormone like factors)
• Multiple myeloma
• Drugs e.g. thiazide diuretics
• Vitamin-D toxicity
• Milk-alkali syndrome
• Sarcoidosis
• Hyperthyroidism
• Addison's disease
• Familial hypocalciuric hypercalcaemia

What are the symptoms of hypercalcaemia?

Hypercalcaemia can present with non-specific symptoms including: polyuria, polydipsia, constipation, nausea, vomiting, depression, confusion, fatigue

The symptoms of hypercalcaemia can be remembered by:
• Bones: Bone pain and fractures
• Stones: Renal stones
• Moans: Depression
• Groans: Abdominal pain

How does the body store calcium?

The body stores calcium in three ways:
• Bone: Stores 99% of total body calcium. Osteoclasts break down bone to release calcium and phosphate whilst osteoblasts incorporate calcium and phosphate into bone.
• Intracellular: Calcium is an important mediator of intracellular signalling
• Extracellular: In the serum approximately 40% is bound to protein (Albumin), 9% ionic complexes and 51% free ions.

What hormones regulate calcium homeostasis?

• Parathyroid hormone: produced by the parathyroid glands. Parathyroid hormone causes an increase in serum calcium by mobilising calcium from bone (increased osteoclast activity), increasing gut absorption, increasing 1α-hydroxylation of Vitamin-D and increasing renal reabsorbtion of calcium. It also increases urinary excretion of phosphate.
• Vitamin-D (1,25-dihydroxyvitamin D3/calcitriol): Results in increased resorption of calcium from bone, increased urinary reabsorbtion of calcium and increased absorption from the GI tract.
• Calcitonin: lowers calcium levels by decreasing bone calcium resorption by limiting osteoclast activity and by increasing renal excretion.

His serum parathyroid levels are 7.2 pmol/ L (<0.8 – 8.5 pmol/ L)

What are the parathyroid glands?

• There are usually 4 glands (2 sets of pairs – superior and inferior) on the posterior aspect of thyroid that secrete parathyroid hormone.
• The superior glands arise from the 4th pharyngeal pouch, close to where the inferior thyroid artery crosses the recurrent laryngeal nerve.

APPLIED SCIENCES

• The inferior glands arise from the 3rd pharyngeal pouch and vary in their position.

How does serum parathyroid hormone and calcium relate to hyperparathyroidism?

	Calcium	Parathyroid hormone
Primary	Elevated	Elevated/ inappropriately normal
Secondary	Reduced/ normal	Elevated
Tertiary	Elevated	Elevated

SUMMARY

Renal calculi can present with severe colicky loin to groin pain and patients with hypercalcaemia are at greater risk of developing renal calculi. Patients with small renal calculi (<10mm) can initially be managed conservatively as the calculi is likely to pass spontaneously.

Calcium levels are regulated by parathyroid hormone, Vitamin-D and to a lesser extent calcitonin. Hypercalcaemia can present with non-specific symptoms and an underlying cause should be sought. In patients with hypercalcaemia and an elevated serum parathyroid hormone the diagnosis is hyperparathyroidism. There are 3 types of hyperparathyroidism: primary, secondary and tertiary.

TOP TIPS

✚ The use of PR diclofenac in renal colic can be highly effective in controlling a patients' pain.

✚ Always remember to correct serum calcium for the patients' albumin levels.

✚ A normal parathyroid level in a patient with hypercalcaemia suggests primary hyperparathyroidism (a normal parathyroid hormone level is inappropriately high in a patient with hypercalcaemia).

APPLIED SCIENCES

1.9 Hyperkalaemia

Scenario

A 75-year-old man with a PMH of stage 3 CKD underwent a Hartmanns procedure for bowel perforation secondary to diverticulitis 2 days ago. He was notably hypotensive during the operation and has had only 200mls of urine output post-operatively. Blood tests taken on admission and 2 days post operatively are shown below:

	On admission	Day 2 post operatively
Urea (2.5 – 6.7 mmol/ L)	9.5 mmol/ L	25 mmol/L
Creatinine (70 – 130 μmol/ L)	150 μmol/ L	310 μmol/ L
Potassium (3.5 – 5 mmol/ L)	5.1 mmol/ L	Haemolysed

What is the definition of Acute Kidney Injury?

Acute kidney injury (AKI) is an abrupt deterioration of kidney function over a short period of time.
It is the inability of the kidney to excrete the nitrogenous and other waste products of metabolism and can develop over the course of a few hours or days.

What is the diagnostic criteria for Acute Kidney Injury?

Introduced by the KDIGO (Kidney Disease: improving global outcome) organisation in 2012, specific criteria exist for the diagnosis of acute kidney injury1.

Acute Kidney Injury can be diagnosed if any one of the following are present:
• Increase in Serum Creatinine by ≥0.3 mg/dl (≥26.5 lmol/l) within 48 hours; or
• Increase in Serum Creatinine to ≥1.5 times baseline, which have occurred within the prior 7 days; or
• Urine volume < 0.5 ml/kg/h for 6 consecutive hours.

How would you initially manage this patient?

The patient should be stabilised following an ABCDE approach with identification and correction of life-threatening haemodynamic parameters. They require IV access with two large-bore cannulas and fluid resuscitation. Catheterisation should be considered to monitor fluid balance and urine output. Regular review and close monitoring of basic physiological parameters is essential including input/output monitoring.

Identification of the underlying cause is key and warrants a thorough history and examination. Any nephrotoxic medications should be discontinued and an USS KUB should be considered to exclude an obstructive cause for his acute kidney injury. Early involovment of the intensive care/nephrology team should be considered as the patient has poor urine output and significant deterioration in their renal function (they may require renal support).

APPLIED SCIENCES

What investigations would you request?

- Bloods: FBC, U&Es, LFTs, clotting profile
- Urine dipstick testing for blood, protein, leucocytes, nitrites and glucose
- ABG to look for metabolic acidosis and bicarbonate level
- ECG to look for changes suggestive of hyperkalaemia
- USS KUB to exclude an obstructive cause of acute kidney injury

Blood tests are sent to a laboratory and an ABG is performed. It shows:

PaO2	14 kPa	(>10 kPa on air)
pH	7.17	(7.35 – 7.45)
PaCO2	4.2 kPa	(4.5 – 6.0 kPa)
HCO3–	10 mmol/ L	(22 – 26 mmol/ L)
BE -	20 mmol/ L	(+/- 2 mmol/ L)
K+	6.9 mmol/ L	(3.5 – 5 mmol/ L)
Na+	137 mmol/ L	(135 – 145 mmol/ L)

What does the ABG show?

It shows a severe metabolic acidosis with attempted respiratory compensation (low CO2). It also shows hyperkalaemia.

Can you name two hormones which affect potassium levels?

Aldosterone: A steroid hormone of the adrenal cortex. Stimulates absorption of sodium in the distal convoluted tubule of the kidney/collecting duct, and several other organs, at the expense of potassium loss into the urine.
Insulin: Stimulates potassium intake into cells, reducing the serum level.

What effect does acidosis have on potassium?

Potassium and H+ are exchanged at the cell membrane, so that an increase of one ion leads to increased exchange with the other. In metabolic acidosis H+ moves into the intra-cellular space therefore in order to maintain electroneutrality potassium is moved into the extracellular space. Thus in acidosis extracellular potassium levels rise.

What effect does urinary flow rate have on potassium secretion?

Increased urianry flow leads to potassium loss – this is one way in which diuretics promote hypokalaemia

What are the ECG changes associated with hyperkalaemia?

- Decreased P wave amplitude
- Tall tented T waves
- Widening of QRS complex
- Sinusoidal waveform
- Ventricular fibrillation and asystole

How would you manage hyperkalaemia?

Most hospitals have local protocols for treatment of hyperkalaemia and treatment depends on the level of hyperkalaemia. Cardiac protection and careful reduction of potassium is key together with investigation and treatment of the underlying cause. An ECG should be performed to assess for any changes associated with hyperkalaemia.

APPLIED SCIENCES

A K+ of >6.5 and any degree of hyperkalaemia with ECG changes requires urgent treatment:
- The patient should be nursed in a monitored bed
- Give 10-20ml 10% IV calcium gluconate which stabilises the myocardium but does not affect potassium level
- To lower K+ give 5-10 units of Insulin in 50mls 50% dextrose over 5-15 minutes and can be repeated (reduces plasma potassium concentration)
- Nebulised salbutamol should be given (reduces plasma potassium concentration)
- Haemodialysis may be required in severe or refractory cases
- The potassium should be rechecked after this initial treatment
- Calcium resonium does not have an immediate effect, it binds potassium in the GI tract reducing the level over days but may be administrated to aid elimination of potassium from the body

Define the term pH?

pH = -Log10(H$^+$)
- pH is the negative logarithm to the base 10 of H$^+$
- It Is a measure of active hydrogen ion activity
- Solutions with a pH less than 7 are acidic and solutions with a pH greater than 7 are basic or alkaline. Pure water has a pH of 7 (neutral).

What are the causes of a metabolic acidosis?

M	Methanol
U	Uraemia (chronic kidney failure)
D	Diabetic ketoacidosis
P	Propylene glycol
I	Infection, Iron, Isoniazid, Inborn errors of metabolism
L	Lactic acidosis
E	Ethylene glycol
S	Salicylates

After initial fluid resuscitation and treatment of his hyperkalaemia he has a repeat ABG which shows the following:

PaO2	15.2 kPa	(>10 kPa on air)
pH	7.18	(7.35 – 7.45)
PaCO2	4.0 kPa	(4.5 – 6.0 kPa)
HCO3–	10 mmol/ L	(22 – 26 mmol/ L)
BE -	21 mmol/ L	(+/- 2 mmol/ L)
K+	6.8 mmol/ L	(3.5 – 5 mmol/ L)
Na+	136 mmol/ L	(135 – 145 mmol/ L)

How would you manage this patient now?

This patient has refractory acidosis and hyperkalaemia. Therefore ITU should be contacted for consideration of acute renal replacement therapy.

What are the relevant indications for acute renal replacement therapy?

- Persistent hyperkalaemia (>6.5mmol/l)
- Severe metabolic acidosis (pH <7.2)
- Refractory pulmonary oedema
- Signs of uraemic encephalopathy
- Signs of uraemic pericarditis

APPLIED SCIENCES

APPLIED SCIENCES

SUMMARY

Acute kidney injury is an abrupt loss of kidney function that is most commonly caused by dehydration and sepsis combined with nephrotoxic drugs, especially following surgery or contrast agents. The causes of acute kidney injury are commonly categorized into prerenal, renal/intrinsic, and postrenal. Severe complications of acute kidney injury include hyperkalaemia and acidosis. Acute dialysis may be required in patiens with refractory hyperkalaemia, severe metabolic acidosis (pH <7.2), refractory pulmonary oedema, signs of uraemic encephalopathy and signs of uraemic pericarditis. 50-60% of patients admitted to ITU have acute renal failure and developing acute renal failure significantly increases length of hospital stay and mortality.

TOP TIPS

➕ Do not forget to stop all nephrotoxic drugs in a patient with an Acute kidney Injury

➕ Medications that are renally excreted should be dose adjusted in patients who develop and acute kidney injury

➕ Always remember to examine for a palpable bladder/ perform a bladder scan in an elderly male patient who develops worsening renal functioning after having a catheter removed *(they are likely to have a degree of prostatic hypertrophy)*.

Further Reading:
1. Thomas M, Davies A, Dawnay A. Acute kidney injury prevention, detection and management of acute kidney injury up to the point of renal replacement therapy. NICE Clinical Guidelines.(August). 2013.
2. Lewington A, Kanagasundaram S. Acute Kidney Injury. The Renal Association, 2011.

1.10 Adrenals

Scenario

A 28-year-old male presents with a longstanding history of palpitations, head-aches, hyperhidrosis and right-sided flank pain.

What hormones are produced by the adrenal glands

Each layer of the adrenal cortex produces a different hormone.

The outermost layer, the zona glomerulosa, produces the mineralocorticoid aldosterone, which plays a critical role in the renin-aldosterone-angiotensin system (RAAS), mainly involved in blood pressure regulation.

Next, the zona fasciculata is responsible for the production of glucocorticoids, such as cortisol, from its cells.

The innermost layer, the zona reticularis, lies adjacent to the adrenal medulla and produces androgens, such as DHEA.

The adrenal medulla is histologically comprised of chromaffin cells (neuroendocrine cells), responsible for the majority of catecholamine production, namely adrenaline and noradrenaline.

What is the function of the glucocorticoid cortisol

Glucose metabolism: gluconeogenesis and inhibition of insulin resulting in hyperglycaemia and glucose intolerance

Protein: Stimulation of uptake of amino acids in liver and protein catabolism in peripheral muscles

Lipids: Lipolysis in adipose tissue

Immune: Supress immunological responses and acts as an anti-inflamatorry

Explain the renin-angiotensin-aldosterone system (RAAS)

Renin is a hormone produced by the juxtaglomerular cells located in the afferent arterioles of the glomeruli of the kidneys

Renin is secreted in response to hypovolaemic states as there is decreased afferent arteriole pressure, low sodium plasma content and stimulation of the beta-1 adrenergic receptor

Increased renin release leads to the conversion of angiotensinogen to angiotensin I

Angiotensin I is converted to angiotensinogen II in the lungs by angiotensin-convering-enzyme (ACE).

Angiotensin II results in aldosterone release.

Moreover, angiotensin II stimulates ADH secretion, sympathetic activity and vasoconstriction.

What are the actions of aldosterone (mineralocorticoid)

Aldosterone promotes sodium and water retention with excretion of potassium in the kidneys

What clinical condition do you think is responsible for the symptoms described above

Phaeochromocytoma

Please describe the underlying pathology of this condition

Phaeochromocytoma is a neuroendocrine tumour of the medulla of the adrenal glands originating in the chromaffin cells which secrete excessive catecholamines.
They are relatively rare affecting 0.05% of the population with a peak incidence between 30 and 50 years2.
Approximately 25% are associated with familial genetic disorders.

You proceed to examine this patient and notice that they have a large goitre of the neck. What inherited syndrome may this patient suffer from and what is the inheritance pattern

Multiple endocrine neoplasia type IIA, it has an autosomal dominant inheritance

What is the classification of MEN

- MEN I
  o Pancreatic islet cell tumour
  o Primary hyperparathyroidism
  o Pituitary adenoma
- MEN II A
  o Phaeochromocytoma
  o Thyroid medullary carcinoma
  o Primary hyperparathyroidism
- Men IIB
  o Phaeochromocytoma
  o Thyroid medullary carcinoma
  o Mucosal neuromas
  o Marfanoid features

SUMMARY

The adrenal glands are important endocrine organs which lie on the supero-medial aspect of the kidneys. The gland is separated into an outer cortex and inner medulla. The cortex produces steroid hormones and is divided into three zones:
The zone glomerulosa produces mineralocorticoids,
The zona fasciulata produces glucocorticoids (cortisol and corticosterone) and the inner zona reticularis produces androgens. As such, the adrenal gland plays a vital part in the renin-angiotensin-aldosterone system. The medulla produces catecholamines which produce a rapid response in the fight or flight response.
A number of tumours can arise from adrenal tissue, in particular phaeochromocytoma, which can form a part of the inherited condition of multiple neuroendocrine neoplasia (type II).

TOP TIPS

➕ Remember the mneumonic **GFR ACD** for the layers of the adrenal glands. The zona glomerulosa produces aldosterone, the zona fasciculata produces cortisol and the zone reticularis produces DHEA and other androgens.

➕ Don't forget the mneumonic **3 P**'s for MEN I and the mneumonic **3 C**'s for MEN IIA *(catecholamines, calcitonin, calcium)*

Further Reading:
1. Munver R, Yates J, Degan M. Surgical and Radiologic Anatomy of the Adrenals. Campbell-Walsh Urology. 11 ed: Elsevier Health Sciences; 2015:1519-1527.
2. Brady M, Ferri F. Phaeochromocytoma. In: Ferri F, ed. Ferri's Clinical Advisor 2017 2017:966-967.

APPLIED SCIENCES

1.11 Blood Groups

Scenario

A 17-year-old girl presents to ED on a cold winter night with lethargy and painful arms and legs. She thinks that her parents may be carriers of a genetic disease and feels that she has been a bit 'chesty' over the past week.

What are the main differentials?

Sickle disease, Raynaud's Disease, fibromyalgia, peripheral neuropathy, influenza

What investigations would you order?

Bloods including FBC (looking for anaemia), blood film (Howell-Jolly bodies), reticulocyte count (sickle cell disease), haemoglobin electrophoresis, U&Es, LFTs, CRP (infection)
CXR – looking for focal consolidation or pulmonary infiltrates
Urinalysis – any sign of urine infection
Consider blood cultures if febrile

What is the genetic basis of sickle cell disease?

It is an autosomal co-dominant (recessive) condition affecting chromosome 11. There is a single amino acid substitution on the beta chain of valine for the normal glumatic acid. This forms a less soluble haemoglobin molecule with reduced red cell survival. Under low oxygen tension, the haemoglobin precipitates causing agglutination.

What are the complications of sickle cell disease?

There are a number of acute and chronic pathologies that those with sickle cell anaemia may suffer.
Patients can develop haemolytic anaemia causing cardiac failure, whilst vaso-occlusive crises cause pain, often in bones, and can lead to organ ischaemic and infarction. Aplastic crisis can result in rapid worsening of symptoms. Sequestration of red cells can cause splenomegaly and hepatomegaly, whilst an acute chest crises is a serious condition which can develop in combination with a vaso-occlusive crises.

What is your management plan in a patient with sickle cell anaemia?

ABCDE – analgesia as per the WHO analgesic ladder with PRN morphine. Oxygen may be required and the patient should be kept warm, in cases IV hydration may be warranted. Blood should be cross-matched and discussion with the haematology team for consideration of transfusion must be undertaken. Antibiotics must be considered if pyrexic In severe cases. For those who are significantly unwell or for those with an acute chest crises intensive care teams should be involved early.

What are the main blood groups

Group ABO system:
• Group A, Group B, Group O and Group AB
• Group A has A antigens on red cells with anti-B antibodies in plasma.
• Group B has B antigens with anti-A antibodies in plasma.
• Group O has no antigens, but has both anti A and anti B antibodies in plasma.

• Group AB has both A and B antigens, but no antibodies

Rhesus system:
• Defined by presence or absence of the Rh-D antigen on the RBC surface governed by 2 alleles which are D & d
• Homozygous dd individuals are Rh-D negative
• The presence of a D allele indicates that the individual is Rh-D positive
• If a Rh-D negative mother comes into contact with Rh-D positive blood from a fetus, the mother is likely to produce antibodies which may cross the placenta
• This causes haemolytic disease of the newborn

The patient receives one unit of blood the following day, however, just after the transfusion has started the patient complains of severe loin pain, is febrile at 39.6 degrees and is pale and clammy. Her HR is 135, BP 96/60mmHg, sats 94%, RR 28. Approximately 25mls of blood have been transfused. What may have happened in this scenario?

This patient is likely to have had a transfusion reaction. It is likely that this is an acute haemolytic transfusion reaction.

What is your management of this situation?

The blood transfusion must be stopped immediately and the line disconnected from the patient. A systematic ABCDE approach is required and you do this whilst simultaneously resuscitating the patient with high-flow oxygen, crystalloid IV fluids to manage hypotension and bloods including an ABG. The laboratory must be informed immediately for analysis of the sample, and critical care input should be sought. Disseminated intravascular coagulation can result following this reaction and this must be monitored for.

How can transfusion reactions be classified?

Transfusion reactions can be classified into immediate and delayed reactions.
The most important reaction to identify is the acute haemolytic reaction, as described above, which is usually due to ABO incompatibility, most commonly due to clerical error. Other acute reactions include a non-haemolytic febrile transfusion reaction, anaphylaxis, transfusion-related acute lung injury, transfusion associated circulatory overload and metabolic abnormalities such as hyperkalaemia and citrate toxicity.

Delayed reactions can include a delayed haemolytic transfusion reaction which may develop over days to weeks, iron overload if repeated transfusions are administered, graft versus host disease and potential infection of a blood-borne virus in unscreened blood.

What is disseminated intravascular coagulation (DIC)

DIC is the pathological activation of the clotting cascade which results in diffuse intra-vascular thrombosis. Once the clotting factors have been consumed this is followed by pathologic activation of the fibrinolytic system and bleeding ensues.

What are the causes of DIC

Infection
Bleeding
Trauma
Burns
Transfusion reaction

APPLIED SCIENCES

Obstetric complication e.g. eclampsia
Liver failure

What signs and symptoms are suggestive of DIC

- Shock and inadequate tissue perfusion
- Bleeding from mucosal membranes
- Petechial rash
- Hypotension
- Tachycardia

What is the management of DIC

Attempt to correct/remove the underlying cause (i.e. treat sepsis), Early involvement of the haematology team who can guide on management strategies which may involve the following:
- Supportive therapy with blood products, especially fresh frozen plasma, platelets and cryoprecipitate
- Low dose heparin (only in selected cases)
- Intensive care team should also be involved
- Newer technologies such as thromboelastography (TEG®) and rotational thromboelastometry (ROTEM®) can guide which specific factors/components need replacing and give rapid results that can be easily repeated at regular intervals2.

SUMMARY

Sickle cell disease is an autosomal co-dominant condition affecting chromosome 11. Complications include painful vasoocclusive crises and haemolytic anaemia. The most important blood group in humans is the ABO system which is coded by 3 alleles. O is the universal RBC donor due to lack of A & B antigens on the surface of the RBC. Blood group AB is the universal RBC recipient due to lack of antibodies in the serum. Knowledge of the Rhesus system is important in Rhesus negative mothers to prevent haemolytic disease of the new born. There are several types of blood transfusion reaction which can be classified as immediate and delayed reactions. Acute haemolytic reactions occur due to ABO incompatibility and are most commonly caused by administrative error. Disseminated intravascular coagulation is characterised by the activation of the clotting cascade by the release of cytokines and tissue factors from damaged tissue. It can be triggered by infections, trauma and transfusion reactions amongst other causes.

TOP TIPS

 DIC is a favourite topic in MRCS exams – ensure a good grasp of the underlying pathophysiology, causes, investigations and treatment

Further Reading:
1. Ferri F. Disseminated Intravascular Coagulation. Ferri's Clinical Advisor 2017 : 5 Books in 1.2017:385-386.
2. Muller MC, Meijers JC, Vroom MB, Juffermans NP. Utility of thromboelastography and/or thromboelastometry in adults with sepsis: a systematic review. Crit Care. 2014;18(1):R30.

1.12 Hypersensitivity

Scenario

You are the surgical SHO on call in Accident & Emergency and you clerk a 16-year-old boy with probable appendicitis. He was previously fit and well with no previous hospital admissions. A&E ask you to come immediately to see him as his "breathing sounds weird" after he had his IV co-amoxiclav. On attendance the patient is tachypnoeic with angioedema and stridor is audible from the end of the bed.

What is your immediate management of this patient

Ensure adequate resources are present therefore shout for help or pull the 'buzzer'. Immediate IM adrenaline 1:1000 (500 micrograms, 0.5ml) with concurrent ABCDE.

What has likely happened to this patient

The patient has an unknown penicillin allergy and has subsequently developed anaphylaxis.

What is anaphylaxis

A severe, life-threatening, generalised or systemic hypersensitivity reaction.

What causes anaphylaxis and who gets it

It is most common in children and young adults, with a slightly higher proportion in females rather than males.
It is commonly caused by foods including nuts, antibiotics (penicillins and cephalosporins), anaesthetic agents such as suxamethonium and bee/wasp stings.

What are the signs and symptoms of anaphylaxis

Airway – Oral/laryngeal oedema, noises of partial upper airway obstruction such as stridor (classically), sensation of throat closing, complete airway occlusion
Breathing – Tachypnoea, wheeze, hoarseness, shortness of breath, cyanosis, respiratory arrest, fatigue
Circulation – hypotension, pallor, clamminess, chest pain, palpitations
Disability – Anxious, sense of impending doom, reduced GCS
Exposure – Skin changes such as urticarial rash, mucosal erythema and swelling

What is the management of anaphylaxis

Stop/remove causative factor (i.e. stop abx infusion)
ABCDE with IM adrenaline 1:1000 (500 micrograms, 0.5ml)
Steroids and antihistamines – 100mg IV hydrocortisone slowly, 10mg chlorphenamine slowly
Fluid challenge and resuscitation– avoid colloids
Early anaesthetic and ENT input if concerned about airway for consideration of tracheal intubation
If airway fully occluded cricothyroidotomy or surgical airway will be indicated

What are the four main types of hypersensitivity reactions

APPLIED SCIENCES

The 4 main types of hypersensitivity reactions are Type I, Type II, Type III and Type IV. Type V is sometimes used as a further distinguishing subtype from Type II, however, is usually included with Type II

What is a type I hypersensitivity reaction

Type I hypersensivity is the typical allergic reaction, including anaphylaxis, atopy and asthma.
It is mediated by IgE antibody and is an immediate reaction that occurs over minutes. Initially the mast cells are sensitised to the antigen when there is an initial exposure and mast cells are 'sensitised' with IgE. On re-exposure to the allergen, crosslinking causes degranulation of mast cells, resulting in the release of vasoactive compounds such as histamine, leukotrienes and prostaglandins. These result in many systemic features, including vasodilatation and smooth muscle contraction, resulting in bronchospasm.

What is a type II hypersensitivity reaction

A Type II hypersensitivity reaction involves antibody production directed towards cell based antigens (extrinsic or intrinsic) within the body. It is mediated mainly by IgG and IgM that on binding to the antigen result in an immune response. A classical example is ABO red cell incompatibility. In this case the red cells will have different antigens, resulting in antibody production against the 'foreign' antigen and the subsequent immune response. Other examples include autoimmune haemolytic anaemia, myasthenia gravis and Graves disease. The latter two examples may also be classified as Type V as the antibodies specifically bind to cell surface receptors. Detection of Type II hypersensitivity reactions can be aided by the use of the direct and indirect Coombs tests.

What is a type III hypersensitivity reaction

A Type III hypersensitivity reaction involves the formation if immune-complexes (antigen-antibody) in response to antigens not bound to cells. Small complexes are deposited in small blood vessels, joints, and glomeruli. These complexes cause an inflammatory response and fix complement. Conditions associated with conditions are serum sickness, post-streptococcal glomerulonephritis and rheumatoid arthritis.

What is a type IV hypersensitivity reaction

A type IV hypersensitivity reaction is delayed, typically occurring over the course of a few days and unlike the others, is cell mediated as opposed to antibody mediated. T helper cells recognise antigen that is presented on an antigen presenting cell, causing the release of cytokines to activate inflammatory cells such as macrophages. This is therefore mediated by T cells. Examples of type IV reactions include contact dermatitis, tuberculosis, type I diabetes and multiple sclerosis.

Give examples of hypersensitivity reactions relevant to surgery

• Assessing asthma in the pre-operative assessment
• Anaphylaxis caused by antibiotics
• Anaphylaxis caused by anaesthetic induction agent
• Grave's disease requiring thyroidectomy
• Myasthenia gravis requiring thymectomy
• Chronic transplant rejection

Type	Clinical syndromes	Mediators	Detail
Type I/Allergy	Anaphylaxis	IgE	Rapid mast cell degranulation with vasoactive mediators
Type 2/Cytotoxic	AIHA, Goodpasture's	IgG, IgM	Antibody binds to antigen on target cells. Test with Coombs test
Type 3/Immune Complex	Serum sickness, Post strep glomerulonephritis	IgG, Complement	Antibody binds to circulating antigen, leading to immune complex
Type 4/Delayed	Contact dermatitis	T cells	T-helper cells activated by an antigen

SUMMARY

Hypersensitivity reactions are a group of important potentially life threatening medical conditions. Early use of adrenaline is a potentially life-saving intervention for anaphylaxis. It is important as a surgeon to be aware of surgically relevant causes for hypersensitivity reactions and their sequelae, some of which may require surgical input if medical management fails.

TOP TIPS

➕ A useful mnemonic for remembering the types of hypersensitivity reaction is ACID:

➕ o Type I – **A**llergic

➕ o Type II – **C**ytotoxic

➕ o Type III – **I**mmune complex deposition

➕ o Type IV – **D**elayed

APPLIED SCIENCES

1.13 Lung Function Tests

Scenario

You are the CT2 in general surgery conducting a pre-operative assessment of an 82-year-old gentleman undergoing elective laparoscopic repair of bilateral inguinal hernia. He has a past medical history of COPD and ischaemic heart disease. You request a pre-op ECG, CXR and lung function tests.

What are the functions of the lung?

Ventilation
  o Oxygenation of blood
  o Removal of CO_2
Acid base balance
Enzyme production most notably angiotensin-converting enzyme (ACE)
Excretion of waste products

Explain and quantify the following lung functions (in a 70kg male)

Total lung capacity (TLC) [TLC=VC+RV]	Volume of air within lungs after maximum inspiration = 6000ml
Tidal volume (TV)	Volume of air in a normal resting breath = 400-600ml
Expiratory reserve volume (ERV)	Volume of air that can be expired from the FRC = 1200ml
Inspiratory reserve volume (IRV)	Volume of air forcibly inspired, over and above the tidal volume = 2500ml
Functional residual capacity (FRC) [FRC=ERV+RV]	Volume of air remaining in the lungs after a normal expiration = 3000ml
Residual volume (RV) [RV=TLC-VC]	Volume of air remaining in lungs after forced expiration = 1200-1500ml
Vital capacity (VC) [VC=IRV+TV+ERV]	The maximum volume expired after a maximum inspiration = 4800ml

Can you draw a spirometry trace of this?

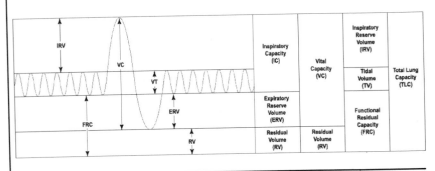

What technique is used to measure residual volume (RV)?

This is an absolute lung volume and therefore cannot be measured by standard spirometry.

Helium dilution technique is one method that uses a closed, rebreathing circuit containing a known amount and concentration of helium. To measure RV the subject starts breathing via the closed circuit after a maximal expiration.

How can you differentiate between obstructive vs restrictive respiratory disease?

The following ratio can be used:
    o FEV1/FVC
FEV is the forced expiratory volume following maximum inspiration
FEV1 is the volume recorded from above during 1st second
<70% (0.7) indicates obstructive disease
>70% (0.7) indicates restrictive disease

Looking at flow loops can also guide on a restrictive or obstructive pattern.

How is oxygen transported in the body?

99% of the bodies oxygen is transported bound to haemoglobin
1% is dissolved in solution

What is haemoglobin composed of?

A haemoglobin molecule consists of four porphyrin rings with a central haem, each of which are attached to a polypeptide chain (globin).
The majority of adult haemoglobin has 2 alpha chains and two beta chains.

Describe the oxygen-haemoglobin dissociation curve

The oxygen haemoglobin dissociation curve is a sigmoid shaped curve that reflects the binding of each molecule to haemoglobin.

What is co-operative binding?

The binding of one oxygen facilitates the binding of the next oxygen molecule. Therefore, haemoglobin binds oxygen with greater affinity, after a subunit has already bound a previous oxygen molecule. The affinity of haemoglobin for the fourth oxygen molecule is as a result of 'co-operative binding' much greater than that of the first.

What is the Bohr Effect?

The Bohr effect is characterised by a shift of the dissociation curve to the right which results in reduced affinity of haemoglobin for oxygen.
This facilitates unloading of oxygen into the tissues at areas of high metabolic activity thus tissues which require oxygen.

What factors cause a right shift of the dissociation curve?

Causes:
• Increased temperature
• Decreased pH
• Increased 2,3 DPG
• Increased $PaCO_2$

APPLIED SCIENCES

Can you draw the oxygen dissociation curve and annotate what shifts the curve left and right?

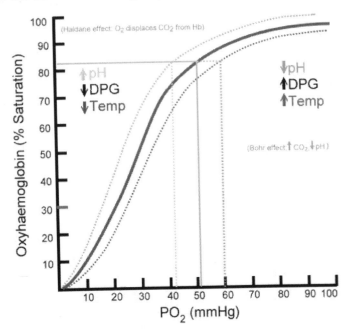

SUMMARY

Lung capacities are important and you could be asked to interpret or explain lung volumes, capacities and significance in the exam. The key pathological differentiation to make is between obstructive and restrictive lung disease. The oxygen dissociation curve relates oxygen saturation and partial pressure of oxygen in blood, and is determined by the haemoglobin affinity for oxygen. It is sigmoidal in shape and can be shifted to the right by increases in pH, CO2, 2,3DPG, exercise and temperature that is known as the Bohr effect.

TOP TIPS

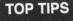 A useful mneumonic for the Bohr effect is **CADET:**

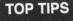 Increased **C**O², Increased **A**cidosis, Increased 2,3 **D**PG, Exercise, Increased **T**emperature

1.14 Neuromuscular Junction

Scenario

You are the SHO in ENT and are seeing a gentleman with a 6-month history of diplopia, hypophonia and tiredness when chewing. He has been referred after unsuccessful medical management.

What is the likely diagnosis?

Myasthenia gravis with referral for consideration of a thymectomy.

What is myasthenia gravis?

Myasthenia gravis is an autoimmune neuromuscular disease resulting in fluctuating muscle weakness and fatigue.

What are the signs and symptoms of myasthenia gravis?

The majority of patients present with eye signs, including diplopia and ptosis, which tends to worsen in bright light and when focussing, for example, reading a book. It can also present with eating difficulties, such as dysphagia and weakness of the muscles of mastication. Patients may have dysarthria or hypophonia whilst the muscles of facial expression can also occasionally be affected. Proximal muscle weakness can also be present. Shortness of breath can occur, if this is severe requiring ventilation the patient is in 'myasthenic crisis'.

What is the pathophysiology of myasthenia gravis?

Myasthenia gravis is an autoimmune condition. Circulating acetylcholine receptor (AChR) antibodies reduce the number of binding sites for ACh binding at the neuromuscular junction. This resulting in skeletal muscle weakness.

Other subtypes of myasthenia gravis are as follows. Muscle-specific tyrosine kinase (MuSK) has a vital role in 'anchoring' AChRs at the post-synaptic plate and those with autoantibodies against MuSK have reduced AChR function and therefore MuSK associated myasthenia gravis. Low-density lipoprotein receptor-related protein (LRP4) is required to activate MuSK therefore autoantibodies to LRP4 also results in myasthenia gravis.

What is a neuromuscular junction?

It is a chemical synapse between the presynaptic membrane of a motor neuron and the postsynaptic membrane of a muscle fibre.

What is an action potential?

An action potential is a transient, regenerative electrical impulse in which the membrane potential rapidly rises to a positive peak which can propagate for long periods along nerve/muscle fibres.

What is the resting membrane potential of a cell?

APPLIED SCIENCES

The resting membrane potential is approximately -70mV at time zero. This is established through the movement of sodium and potassium ions via sodium-potassium pumps. For every 3 sodium ions moved out, 2 potassium ions move in, hence creating a negative gradient. During this time the voltage gated ion channels are closed.

How does cellular depolarisation occur?

When a stimulus is applied, the voltage gated ion channels open, causing a rapid influx of sodium ions which causes the cell interior to become positively charged and it depolarises. The cell membrane then repolarises via the efflux of potassium ions down their concentration gradient. This causes a slight episode of hyperpolarisation due to excess potassium efflux along the concentration gradient, however, this is quickly rectified via the regular sodium-potassium pump

What is the 'all or nothing principle'?

The all or nothing principle states that the strength a neuron or muscle fibre responds to a stimulus is independent of the strength of the applied stimulus. As long as the stimuli allows the membrane to reach its threshold potential, approximately -50mV, an action potential will be generated and propagated and the resulting tissue will provide a maximal response. If the membrane does not reach the threshold potential, no action potential will be generated and there will be no response.

Describe the physiology at the neuromuscular junction?

Upon arrival of an action potential at the presynaptic terminal, voltage gated calcium channels open and calcium flows into the presynaptic neuron. This causes the release of acetylcholine via vesicles at the pre-synaptic terminal. The acetylcholine diffuses across the synaptic cleft and binds to acetylcholine receptors at the post-synaptic membrane. The acetylcholine is then release and broken down by acetylcholinesterase. This is utilised in the medical treatment of myasthenia gravis by increasing the amount of acetylcholine in the synaptic cleft by using acetylcholinesterase inhibitors.

What is the anatomy of skeletal muscle?

The basic cell of skeletal muscle is the myocyte. Myocytes are surrounded by a fascia called the endomysium. Groups of myocytes are arranged in bundles, called fascicles. The fascicles are surrounded by perimysium, a form of connective tissue. Groups of fascicles are arranged into muscle, which is surrounded by the final fascial layer, the epimysium.

What is the microscopic anatomy of skeletal muscle?

The basic functional unit of a myocyte is a myofibril. The myocyte is densely packed with myofibrils which are formed into chains within a myocyte. The myofibrils are made up of organised repeating units called sarcomeres which consist of smaller filaments called myofilaments of which there are 2 types, thick and thin filaments. Thick filaments are mainly comprised of myosin and thin filaments of actin. The highly organised sarcomeres gives rise to the term 'striated muscle'. Troponin and tropomyosin are two other proteins involved in muscle contraction.

The cell membrane of a myocyte is known as the sarcolemma and has transverse (t) tubules which extend the membrane into the muscle cell. The sarcoplasmic reticulum (SR) is a specialised form of endoplasmic reticulum and forms a network around the myofibrils. This network is bookended by two terminal cisternae (specialised regions of the

SR) which are associated with a single t-tubule. This sarcoplasmic reticulum serves as a reservoir for calcium ions, and when an action potential spreads through the t-tubule, this stimulates the sarcoplasmic reticulum to release calcium and foster a contraction.

What is a sarcomere?

A sarcomere is the segment between two neighbouring z-lines. The sacromere contains multiple sections, known as the I-band, A-band, H-band and M-line. The I-band is simply thin filaments alone. The A-band is both thick and thin filaments, including one thick filament of full length. The H-band contains only thick filaments. The M-line is within the H-band and contains the connecting cytoskeleton proteins, there are no cross bridges in this region.

What is the process of muscle contraction?

The process by which an action potential results in muscular contraction is known as 'excitation contraction coupling'.

When an action potential is propagated along the sarcolemma down the t-tubules this causes the stored calcium in the sarcoplasmic reticulum to be released. The calcium binds to troponin C on actin that interacts with troponin I. This causes the movement of tropomyosin to expose the myosin binding sites on actin. The myosin binds to actin forming a cross-link. The release of phosphate causes the 'power stroke' pulling the two sarcomeres closer together (sliding filament theory) and ADP is also released. ATP then binds to the cross bridge which releases the bond between actin and myosin. The ATP is hydrolysed to ADP energising the myosin for the next contraction.

High levels of calcium cause calcium channels to close and calcium is pumped back into the SR (active process therefore requiring ATP). As the cytoplasmic level of calcium falls calcium is released from Troponin C and tropomyosin blocks the myosin binding site.

The myosin pulls the actin filament about 11nm during a power stroke.

APPLIED SCIENCES

SUMMARY

Myasthenia gravis is a neurological condition associated with fatigability. It is treated with acetylcholinterase inhibitors and in certain cases thymectomy, especially if a thymoma is present. Action potentials stimulate a muscular contraction through the release of calcium from the sarcoplasmic reticulum and the subsequent cross-linking of actin and myosin, creating a power stroke. Cardiac muscle is involuntary and is stimulated via constantly depolarising pacemaker cells, whereas skeletal muscle is under voluntary control and stimulated via somatic neurons.

TOP TIPS

Do not forget the importance of essential ions in the routine functioning of the nervous system. Consequently large changes out of the reference ranges for sodium, potassium and calcium can have fatal consequences.

1.15   Intracranial Pressure

Scenario

A normally fit and well 49 year old gentleman presents with a sudden onset severe neck pain with an associated headache that he describes as the worst headache of his life. Furthermore he complains of marked nausea. He is normally well and does not suffer from headaches.

What is your differential diagnosis?

- Subarachnoid haemorrhage (SAH)
- Non-sinister headache (migraine, tension, cluster)
- Stroke (haemorrhagic or thrombotic)
- Meningitis

What would your initial management plan consist of?

- ABCDE approach with subsequent full history and examination
- Oxygen, IV access, routine bloods including a cross match and clotting studies (ensure not on anti-thrombotics)
- Routine observations including Glasgow Coma Score
- CT brain

A non-contrast CT brain is performed. Describe what you see in the image.

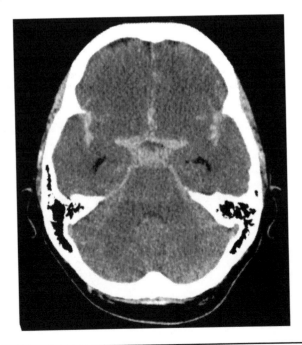

This axial non contrast CT scan reveals widespread subarachnoid blood.

If the CT was normal what would your next step be?

The patient would require a lumbar puncture 12 hours after onset of symtpoms looking for blood/xanthochromia

In light of the CT findings who must be contacted?

• Neurosurgical team/referral hub
• Discussion with radiology regarding further imaging +/- interventional options should be considered (note often the neurosurgical team will discuss directly with a neuro interventional radiologist)

What are the causes of a subarachnoid haemorrhage (SAH)?

• Saccular (Berry) aneurysm (approximately 85%) often in the region of the Circle of Willis
• Non-aneurysmal haemorrhages (approximately 10%)
• Arteriovenous malformations and vertebral artery dissection (approximately 5%)
• Traumatic

Sometimes these patients will develop signs of raised intracranial pressure (ICP) which reduces cellular perfusion and results in cell death. Are you aware of an equation for cerebral perfusion pressure?

Cerebral perfusion pressure = mean arterial pressure – intracranial pressure

What is regarded as a normal ICP?

Normal ICP is 5 - 15 mmHg

Can you explain the Monro-Kellie doctrine?

The Monro-Kellie doctrine states that an increase in the volume of any of the calvarial contents (brain tissue, blood, CSF, or brain fluids) must be accompanied by a decrease in the volume of another component, or intracranial pressure will increase markedly because the bony calvarium rigidly fixes the total cranial volume.

Can you draw a diagram to represent the Monro-Kellie doctrine?

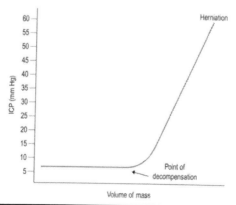

What are some key complications following SAH?

- Raised ICP
- Decreased GCS and neurological activity
- Seizure activity
- Vasospasm
- Cardiac arrest
- Re-bleeding
- Death
- Long term reduced neurological function or complications such as epilepsy

In this case further imaging revealed a berry aneurysm was found, how would this likely be managed?

Rebleeding is associated with high mortality and poor prognosis thus the aneurysm should be managed using either endovascular or surgical options (essentially coiling or clipping)

Prior to intervention if the patient developed signs of raised ICP how can this be managed?

- Nurse with head up at around 30 degrees
- Ensure pain is controlled
- Sedation
- Intubation and control of ventilation to both maintain oxygenation and prevent hypercapnia
- Aim for normovolaemia
- Maintain a CPP of over 80mmHg (hypotensive periods must be avoided)
- Manage seizures
- Consider osmotic diuretic such as mannitol
- May need insertion of Intraventricular drain
- Ideally insert ICP bolt

The patient has had their aneurysm managed, are you aware of any specific management post SAH utilised in the ICU?

Cerebral vasospasm following SAH and can result in further ischaemic insult. This occurs around 7-10 days post SAH. 'Triple H therapy', although controversial, is used in some units as an attempt to prevent this. This therapy involves achieving hypertension, hypervolemia, hemodilution. As it is not without risk some have now moved to euvolaemia with induced hypertension, however further evidence is needed to clearly demonstrate the optimum therapy.

SUMMARY

The pressure-volume relationship between ICP, volume of CSF, blood, and brain tissue, and cerebral perfusion pressure (CPP) is known as the Monro-Kellie doctrine or the Monro-Kellie hypothesis.
The Monro-Kellie hypothesis states that the cranial compartment is incompressible and that the volume inside the cranium is fixed. The cranium and its constituents (blood, CSF, and brain tissue) create a state of volume equilibrium, such that any increase in volume of one of the cranial constituents must be compensated by a decrease in volume of another.

The principal buffers for increased volumes include CSF and, to a lesser extent, blood volume. These buffers respond to increases in volume of the remaining intracranial constituents. For example, an increase in lesion volume (e.g. epidural hematoma) will be compensated by the downward displacement of CSF and venous blood. These compensatory mechanisms are able to maintain a normal ICP for any change in volume less than approximately 100–120 mL.

TOP TIPS

➕ Intracranial haemorrhage is a common clinical presentation and early imaging to establish a diagnosis is imperative.

➕ Remember that the skull is a 'fixed box' and urgent neurosurgical advice should be sought.

➕ Keep in mind the non-surgical methods for reducing ICP in order to 'buy time' before radiological/surgical interventions.

APPLIED SCIENCES

1.16 Coagulopathies

Scenario

You are seeing a patient in pre-assessment clinic prior to an elective total knee replacement surgery. During your consultation you discover that the patient is taking warfarin.

How would you manage this patient?

A full history and examination forms part of pre-assessment. In this case, the indication for warfarin therapy should be ascertained and a risk/benefit analysis regarding the perioperative management of their thrombosis risk performed. Hospitals often have their own policies for warfarin bridging around the time of surgery, and a common rule of thumb is that the INR should be less than 1.5 to safely proceed with surgery. Post-operatively the warfarin can be re-started either the evening after surgery or the following day (as long as there is no concern regarding haemostasis is adequate.

If in doubt, it is recommended to clarify perioperative management (which may include, for example, bridging low-molecular weight heparin) with a haematologist.

Briefly describe the coagulation cascade

The coagulation cascade refers to an organised cascade of proteins which ultimately facilitates the conversion of fibrinogen into fibrin. Fibrin is required in order for platelets to form an effective clot. The cascade is traditionally split into 3 distinct pathways (though this is now recognised as an over-simplified paradigm).

• The intrinsic pathway- begins with 'contact activation' in which a charged surface activates factor XII, which in turn activates a sequence of clotting factors. The intrinsic pathway converges with the extrinsic pathway with the activation of factor X.

• The extrinsic pathway- when circulating factor VII comes into contact with tissue factor it is activated to form VIIa, which promotes the activation of factor X.

• The common pathway- is the final common pathway of the intrinsic and extrinsic pathways. It culminates with the conversion of prothrombin to thrombin, which in turn converts fibrinogen to fibrin.

What is the mechanism of action of warfarin?

Warfarin inhibits the synthesis of the vitamin-K dependant clotting factors. Specifically, its main effects are on the synthesis of clotting factors II, VII, IX, and X, as well as proteins C and S.

What effect does warfarin have on prothrombin time and activated partial thromboplastin time and why?

Warfarin primarily affects the extrinsic arm of the coagulation cascade. This will manifest as a prolonged PT and normal APTT.

Can warfarin cause a hypercoagulable state?

Yes. Warfarin exerts its effects on proteins C and S quicker than its effects on the clotting factors. This results in a temporary procoagulant effect.

List some factors which can potentiate the effects of warfarin

- P450 enzyme inducers such as amiodarone
- Liver disease
- Drugs that displace warfarin from albumin such as NSAIDS
- Antiplatelet medications
- Alcohol excess

What is Virchow's triad?

Virchow's triad includes endothelial injury, alterations to blood flow, and hypercoagulability. It describes three factors precipitating thrombus formation.

List some risk factors for developing postoperative venous thromboembolism

The risk factors for developing post-operative VTE can be divided into patient-related and procedure-related factors.

Patient factors include:
- Increased age
- Increased BMI
- Personal or family history of VTE
- Malignancy
- Medications such as the oral contraceptive pill
- Dehydration
- Pregnancy
- Smoking

Procedural factors include:
- Lower limb or pelvic orthopaedic surgery
- Prolonged surgical time
- Pneumoperitoneum (at laparoscopy)
- Postoperative immobility

You move on to review your next patient. They are taking aspirin and clopidogrel. What are the mechanisms of action of these drugs?

Both function as antiplatelet drugs. Aspirin irreversibly inhibits cyclooxygense (COX) enzymes 1 and 2. As such (via COX 1 inhibition) it affects the production of prostaglandins and thromboxanes from arachidonic acid. Clopidogrel is an irreversible adenosine diphosphate (ADP) receptor antagonist. By preventing ADP from binding its platelet receptor, it inhibits platelet aggregation.

Your FY1 is also in the preassessment clinic. She is assessing a patient listed for elective hip arthroplasty who is taking aspirin for primary prevention. She asks your advice about how to manage his aspirin perioperatively?

It is always advisable to check if the hospital has a local policy, and many will have well-established local guidance. There is evidence of aspirin increasing bleeding complications at major orthopaedic procedures such as total hip replacement surgery. As such, many units would advise stopping taking the aspirin approximately 5 days preoperatively to minimise these risks.

Imagine instead that the patient is taking aspirin as a result of having a cardiac stent recently fitted following myocardial infarction. How would your advice change?

This would of course change the risk/benefit analysis of stopping aspirin perioperatively. Particularly with bare metal stents, stopping antiplatelet medication increases the risk of stent occlusion.

More importantly however, given that this patient is being preassessed for elective surgery, this history should prompt a review as to whether the patient is fit to proceed or whether the procedure should be delayed or even cancelled.

What is a NOAC?

NOAC stands for new (or novel) oral anticoagulant. It refers to a new group of anticoagulant medications which directly inhibit activated factor X (Xa). The most widely used in the UK are rivaroxaban and apixaban.

You notice that your final preassesment patient is young for a total knee replacement. He tells you his knee problems result from having bled into his knee a number of times, often spontaneously or after negligible trauma. What might be going on in this situation and what preassessment issues does this raise?

This gentleman suffers from haemophilia, of which haemophilic arthropathy is a well-recognised sequela. His haemophilia will require managing perioperatively and this should be via a multidisciplinary approach with the haematological, anaesthetic and surgical teams. It is likely to involve repeated monitoring and infusion of the deficient clotting factor (VIII or IX, depending on subtype of haemophilia).

SUMMARY

The ageing population and increasing prevalence of patients with multiple comorbidities means that surgical patients- both elective and emergency- are frequently taking antiplatelet or anticoagulant medication. These have obvious implications intraoperatively and necessitate careful perioperative management. Surgeons should be familiar with their pharmacology and confident in managing their use around the time of surgery. Perhaps even more importantly however, surgeons should be alert for the cases requiring more complex perioperative management (such as reversal, or bridging therapy) and be quick to involve the relevant specialty where necessary.

APPLIED SCIENCES

TOP TIPS

➕ When describing VTE risk factors, the example used above *(patient- and procedure-related factors)* is just one example. Other potential divisions are congenital versus acquired risk factors, or preoperative versus intraoperative versus postoperative factors.

➕ The preassessment clinic has a vital role in determining fitness for surgery. If unsure, have a low threshold for discussion with the relevant team.

➕ Even in a physiology/basic science station, patient safety is always paramount.

APPLIED SCIENCES

2 PATHOLOGY

PATHOLOGY

2.1 Clostridium Difficile

Scenario

You are the on-call CT2 for general surgery. You are called to see a 78 year old patient who has been in hospital receiving intravenous antibiotics for 8 days. They have developed bloody diarrhoea with mucus, and have become slightly hypotensive and tachycardic. The patient is comfortable. You have already washed your hands, introduced yourself and explained what you are going to do.

What is your differential diagnosis?

Clostridium difficile ("C diff") diarrhoea (due to the preceding antibiotics)
Viral gastroenteritis
Ischaemic colitis
Inflammatory bowel disease

How would you manage this patient?

The patient should be managed with an ABCDE approach. Intravenous access should be gained and appropriate blood tests sent. The tachycardia and hypotension should prompt an intravenous fluid challenge with an appropriate crystalloid. The response to the challenge should be assessed and further fluid resuscitation planned accordingly. The fluid balance chart and stool chart should be taken into account when calculating maintenance fluid requirements thereafter. He should be catheterised to measure urine output accurately.

The indication to continue the previous antibiotics should be considered and the antibiotic changed or stopped under microbiology guidance if safe to do so. A stool sample for MC&S and C.Diff toxin should be sent.

The definitive treatment would be guided by the severity of the infection and is likely to be outlined in a local guideline. Appropriate antibiotics could be either intravenous vancomycin or oral metronidazole. In addition, anti-diarrhoeals and opiates (which slow gut transit) should be avoided.

In very rare cases, urgent surgical management including subtotal or even total colectomy may be required.

What investigation would aid your diagnosis?

- Bloods:
    - Full blood count and C reactive protein as markers of inflammation
    - Urea and electrolytes to assess for metabolic abnormality secondary to dehydration (e.g. acute kidney injury or hyperkalaemia).
- Stool sample for MC+S and C.Diff toxin (ELISA)
- Blood cultures
- ABG (for lactate)
- AXR +/- erect CXR if any concerns regarding potential perforation
- CT abdomen/pelvis if required, looking for mucosal thickening or pseudomembranous colitis
- Flexible sigmoidoscopy/colonoscopy to take biopsies and visualise the grey/yellow plaques of pseudomembranous colitis

PATHOLOGY

What type of pathogen is Clostridium difficile and how does it cause colitis?

It is a gram positive spore-forming anaerobe. It releases enterotoxins A and B. The toxins cause acute inflammation in the mucosa of the colon leading to its destruction. The pseudomembranes (hence 'pseudomembranous colitis') are grey/yellow plaques formed from acute neutrophil infiltration, exudate and sloughed mucosa.

How is Clostridium difficile transmitted?

The faeco-oral route is usually responsible for the spread of C. Diff. It is often a hospital-acquired infection, and strict isolation procedures are followed in confirmed or suspected cases.

What are the risk factors for acquiring Clostridium difficile?

- Antibiotic use (e.g. clindamycin, cephalosporins, co-amoxiclav)
- Increased age
- Increased length of hospital stay
- Contact with other patients with C.Diff
- Proton pump inhibitors
- Poor hand hygiene

How do antibiotics predispose a patient to Clostridium difficile colitis?

Systemic antibiotics disrupt the normal gut flora. This allows (and encourages) increased growth of resistant bacteria such as Clostridium difficile.

How do you diagnose severe Clostridium difficile colitis?

The presence of one or more of the following criteria suggests a severe colitis:
- White cell count >15x109/L
- Creatinine >50% above baseline
- Temperature >38.5 degrees Celcius
- Clinical/radiological evidence of severe colitis (toxic megacolon, rising lactate)

What complications can arise from Clostridium difficile colitis?

- Fulminant colitis
- Paralytic ileus
- Toxic megacolon
- Colonic perforation
- Multi-organ failure & death (e.g. from dehydration)

What percentage of patients will get a recurrence of Clostridium difficile after their first treatment with either metronidazole or vancomycin?

Approximately 20% will relapse having completed treatment for a first case of Clostridium difficile. Those that relapse are subsequently at risk for further relapses.

PATHOLOGY

SUMMARY

Any patient displaying signs of haemodynamic instability should be assessed with an ABCDE approach and assumed to be unstable until proven otherwise. In assessing a patient with diarrhoea, as in this scenario, it is prudent to be mindful not only of dehydration but the metabolic abnormalities which can result from it. If Clostridium difficile is suspected, it is important to bear in mind the need to isolate the patient alongside any other local infection control procedures. It is also important to bear in mind that Clostridium difficile is associated with significant morbidity, particularly amongst the elderly, and that it does have a number of serious sequelae.

TOP TIPS

➕ Alcohol based washes are not bactericidal to C difficile. This should be borne in mind when hand-washing before and particularly after dealing with a patient with suspected C diff: soap and water and not alcohol gel!

➕ Bloody diarrhoea, as in this scenario, only accounts for approximately 5% of presentations of Clostridium difficile. The usual presentation is of profuse watery diarrhoea.

PATHOLOGY

2.2 Inflammation

Scenario

You are called to the emergency department minors to see a 25-year-old male with a lump on his arm. One week ago he recalls an insect bite at this location. The lump is approximately 4cm in maximal diameter, warm, tender and fluctuant. There is a degree of surrounding erythema.

What is your diagnosis?

The history is strongly suggestive of an abscess.

How would you manage this patient?

Patients with abscesses can become septic, and thus management should begin with a rapid ABCDE assessment to ensure stability. Blood should be drawn for inflammatory markers, full blood count, lactate and blood cultures. Allergy status should be determined and appropriate antibiotics commenced according to local policy. The case should be discussed with a senior team member, as incision and drainage in theatre is likely to be indicated.

What investigation would aid your diagnosis?

• Full blood count and CRP
• Blood cultures
• Lactate
• Blood sugsr: diabetes is associated with abscess formation
• Ultrasound: Can be useful if the presence of a collection is uncertain. Can also demonstrate the size and position of the collection in order to help plan surgery. In certain situations, such as if the site in question was about an injection site in a patient with history of intravenous drug use, can be useful to rule out any communication with the vessels.
• MRI: if there is concern about the depth of an abscess, or communication with other structures, MRI can be used to accurately delineate the abscess.

What is an abscess?

An abscess is a contained, localised collection of pus within tissue, surrounded by granulation/fibrous tissue.

What is pus?

Pus is a viscous liquid containing inflammatory proteins, neutrophils, and debris from dead/dying micro-organisms and degraded neutrophils.

What are the cardinal signs characteristic of acute inflammation?

Heat, redness, swelling and pain (or calor, rubor tumor and dolor respectively). Impaired function is often included as the fifth cardinal sign.

What are the stages of acute inflammation?

• Release of proinflammatory mediators

PATHOLOGY

- Local vasodilation and increased blood flow
- Increased vascular permeability leading to fluid exudate
- Leucocyte extravasation (diapedesis) (primarily neutrophils)
- Neutrophil phagocytosis
- Resolution or formation of pus or granulation or progression to chronic inflammation

Which cell types are present in chronic inflammation?

The principal inflammatory cells involved in chronic inflammation are macrophages and lymphocytes.

What are the causes of chronic inflammation?

- Infection e.g. TB, syphilis
- Toxins e.g. asbestosis
- Autoimmune disease e.g. rheumatoid arthritis
- Immunodeficiency e.g. HIV, prolonged steroid use
- Malignancy
- Malnutrition
- Idiopathic e.g. sarcoidosis

SUMMARY

Inflammation is a complex physiological process. It usually occurs due to an insult which can be physical (e.g. mechanical), biological (infection by a pathogen), environmental (e.g. temperature), or in the case of autoimmune disease may be part of 'normal' physiology. There are a number of outcomes to an episode of inflammation including complete resolution, scarring and fibrosis, or progression to chronic inflammation.

TOP TIPS

 Acute inflammation *(characterised as occurring from minutes after the insult through to days)* and chronic inflammation *(days to weeks)* are often described as two separate entities. In vivo they often overlap.

 Biochemical evidence of an acute inflammatory reaction includes increased acute phase protein concentrations *(e.g. CRP)*, increased erythrocyte sedimentation rate, and neutrophilia in the full blood count.

PATHOLOGY

2.3 Tuberculosis

> ### Scenario
>
> An 80-year-old lady who was admitted earlier in the day with a left sided neck of femur fracture has a chest radiograph as part of her pre-operative work up. It shows a small rounded lesion in the left upper lobe.

What is your differential diagnosis?

Tuberculosis
Fungal infection
Malignancy
Benign pulmonary nodule
Sarcoidosis

How would you manage this patient?

This patient has sustained a significant injury and should be initially assessed with the ABCDE protocol, identifying and addressing any haemodynamic abnormalities. A full history including past medical history, drug history, family history and social history is required. Specifically to this case travel history, smoking history, vaccination history and possible TB exposure is pertinent. Detailed cardiorespiratory examination should be performed, both to aid in the diagnosis of the lung lesion and to inform on anaesthetic fitness. In the social history, it is vital to determine the pre-injury mobility as this may affect the surgical management.

What investigation would aid your diagnosis of the chest lesion?

- Full blood count and CRP for markers of infection
- Arterial blood gas analysis if there is any sign of hypoxaemia
- Sputum samples sent for acid-fast bacilli smear and culture
- Interferon gamma release assays for TB
- Blood cultures
- CT thorax- will be able to further characterise the lesion

What are the clinical features of pulmonary TB?

- Productive cough
- Fevers and night sweats
- Weight loss
- Malaise
- Haemoptysis
- Pleuritic pain
- Pleural effusion

What is the pathophysiology of secondary TB?

Secondary TB is usually a result of reactivation of latent TB due to reduced host immunity, but it may also be due to reinfection. Typically it develops in the upper lobes of the lungs. TB causes a hypersensitivity reaction leading to tissue destruction and cavitation with formation of caseating granulomas.

What is a Ghon complex?

A Ghon complex is the combination of a Ghon focus (a calcified lung lesion, usually at the pleural surface) and associated lymphadenopathy.

How are sputum samples analysed for TB?

Microscopy of a smear of sputum stained with the Zeihl-Neelsen stain (stains acid-fast bacilli) on microscopy and culture in Lowenstein-Jensen media.

What is miliary tuberculosis?

Miliary TB refers to the widespread dissemination of tuberculosis characterised by numerous small lesions throughout the lungs and a number of other extrapulmonary sites, especially the liver and spleen.

What are Pott's disease and lupus vulgaris?

Both are named, extrapulmonary sites of tuberculosis infection. Pott's disease refers to tuberculosis of the spine. This is usually secondary to a source of infection elsewhere and is now rare in developed countries. Lupus vulgaris is the most common tuberculous skin infection and is a painful, nodular plaque most often found on the face or neck.

There are a number of extrapulmonary manifestations of TB and these occur more frequently in the immunosuppressed.

What are the Mantoux and Heaf tests?

They are both tests which can be used to test for active infection or previous vaccination. A protein derivative of tuberculin, a protein extracted from Mycobacterium tuberculosis is used to stimulate a delayed hypersensitivity reaction. In the Mantoux test, a sample is injected into the dermis, and the diameter of any resulting papule measured at 72 hours. In the Heaf test, multiple shallow punctures in the skin are inoculated, with the number of papules present at 72 hours determining a positive or negative result.

Describe the Coombs and Gell classification of hypersensitivity reactions.

Type	Alternative nomenclature	Principal mediator	Summary
1	Allergic/Anaphylactic	Immunoglobulin E	Antigen activates IgE expressed on mast cells causing histamine release
2	Cytotoxic (antibody-mediated)	Immunoglobulins M and G, complement cascade	Complement-mediated formation of the membrane attack complex against a cell perceived as exogenous (due to an antigen expressed on its membrane.

PATHOLOGY

| 3 | Immune complex mediated | Immunoglobulin G, neutrophils | Antibody-antigen complexes initiate acute inflammatory response |
| 4 | Delayed | T lymphocytes | Inflammatory response in response to a specific antigen, stimulated by pre-sensitised immune cells. |

SUMMARY

Tuberculosis, caused by Mycobacterium tuberculosis, remains a significant source or mortality and morbidity worldwide, and there is increasing evidence of multiple drug-resistant strains. There is also evidence of increasing incidence in certain parts of the United Kingdom, where it remains a notifiable disease. The treatment of tuberculosis is usually a prolonged course of multiple synergistic antibiotics.

TOP TIPS

· The classification for hypersensitivity reactions examined in this scenario can be recalled using the mnemonic 'ACID', for 'allergic', 'cytotoxic', 'immune-complex' and 'delayed'.

2.4 Gangrene

Scenario

You are a CT2 trainee in a vascular clinic. You see a 65 year old patient who has been referred to the clinic because of a black, well defined lesion affecting his 2nd and 3rd toes on the right foot. The toes are insensate and noticeably colder than on the contralateral side. He is diabetic and has a 50 pack-year smoking history. The patient is haemodynamically stable with no signs of sepsis.

What is the most likely diagnosis?

Dry Gangrene is the most likely diagnosis.

How would you manage this patient?

There are a number of management options. The least invasive is expectant management, which will end with autoamputation of the affected tissues. This is only a viable treatment option in non-vital tissues. Depending on the extent of the ishchaemia, open or endovascular revascularisation may be an option. Finally, surgical debridement +/- amputation of the affected areas should be considered. If there is any evidence of infection, antibiotics should be commenced in line with the local protocol.

Describe the differences between wet and dry gangrene

Dry gangrene is due to critical interruption of the arterial supply and is the end-point of untreated peripheral arterial disease. There is no superimposed infection, the affected area is cold, shrunken, odourless, haemosiderin-stained and tends to have a clear line of demarcation between viable and non-viable tissue.

Wet gangrene is ischaemic necrosis with superimposed infection. It usually has an ill-defined edge with evidence of ulceration and skin blistering. It is painful, malodorous, and if untreated will spread proximally. Wet gangrene is caused by blockage of both venous and arterial systems.

What are the causes of gangrene?

Peripheral vascular disease, embolus/thrombosis causing acute limb ischaemia, Raynaud's disease, thromboangiitis obliterans and other vasculitidies, ergot poisoning, vessel injury secondary to extreme cold/heat/trauma/pressure (e.g. frostbite), and drug induced (e.g warfarin necrosis).

As part of your clinic assessment you perform ABPIs. Please explain this test.

ABPI stands for ankle-brachial pressure index. It is performed by measuring the systolic blood pressure at the brachial artery, and comparing this to the systolic pressure at the ankle (using a Doppler probe). The 'ankle' value is then divided by the 'brachial' value to give a ratio.

A normal result is 1. If the result is >1.3 then this suggests erroneously high reading at the ankle due to heavy calcification of the vessels. A result is between 0.9-0.5 suggests

PATHOLOGY

peripheral arterial disease and is likely to correlate with symptomatic intermittent claudication. Values between 0.5-0.3 usually correlate with rest pain due to significant limb ischaemia and values <0.2 are compatible with critical ischaemia, gangrene and ulceration.

What are the risk factors for chronic limb ischaemia?

The risk factors can be classified as either modifiable or non-modifiable.

Modifiable risk factors include:
o Smoking
o Hypertension
o Glycaemic control
o Hyperlipidaemia
o Poor exercise.
The non-modifiable risk factors include:
o Increased age
o Male sex
o Positive family history
o Past medical history

What are the signs of acute limb ischaemia?

Acute limb ischaemia is caused by sudden perturbation to the blood supply of a limb. The symptoms are classically described as 'the 6 P's':
o Pain
o Pallor
o Pulselessness
o 'Perishingly' cold
o Paraesthesia
o Paralysis

You receive a call from the FY1 covering the ward. One of your patients has developed a painful, rapidly spreading cellulitis. The centre has become discoloured and started to blister, with palpable subcutaneous emphysema.

What are you worried might be the diagnosis?

This must be assumed to be necrotising fasciitis until proven otherwise. Other differentials include cellulitis, erysipelas, and pumphigus/pemphigoid, amongst others.

What is necrotising fasciitis?

Necrotising fasciitis is a rapidly-spreading infection causing necrosis of the subcutaneous tissues as it spreads along the fascial planes. It is more common in the immunosuppressed. Though historically associated with group A β-haemolytic streptococcus, necrotising fasciitis is commonly polymicrobial. It carries high rates of morbidity and mortality.

How would you manage this patient?

Necrotising fasciitis is a surgical emergency. ABCDE assessment should be completed, ensuring large bore IV access is gained and fluid resuscitation with an appropriate crystalloid commenced. Broad spectrum intravenous antibiotics and analgesia should be administered. The appropriate senior surgical colleague should be contacted urgently. An emergency theatre should be booked, the emergency anaesthetic team notified, and the HDU/ITU teams notified. Necrotising fasciitis mandates urgent radical debridement.

What is Meleney's gangrene?

A form of gangrene occurring around post-operative wounds due to synergistic bacteria. It causes extensive soft tissue necrosis and ulceration.

What is Fournier gangrene?

Fournier gangrene refers to necrotising fasciitis of the perineum. Like necrotising fasciitis elsewhere, it is a rapidly spreading, life-threatening infection necessitating emergency resuscitation, broad-spectrum antibiosis, and radical surgical debridement.

SUMMARY

Gangrene refers to a broad group of conditions characterised by ischaemic necrosis of tissues with or without superimposed infection. Though the examples in this scenario have been peripheral, the term can be applied to any ischaemic tissue, such as mesenteric ischaemia causing gangrene of the small bowel. Depending on the type of gangrene, management differs vastly. For example, isolated distal dry gangrene can be managed expectantly, awaiting autoamputation over a period of months. In contrast, 'gas' gangrene secondary to clostridium infection and necrotising fasciitis are surgical emergencies associated with high morbidity and mortality.

TOP TIPS

 The order of the numerator and denominator in measuring ankle-brachial pressure indices can be extrapolated from the abbreviation: ABPI- 'ankle' before 'brachial'.

PATHOLOGY

2.5 | **Peptic Ulceration**

Scenario

An 80-year-old patient presents to the emergency department with sudden-onset upper abdominal pain. He is a lifelong smoker and has recently completed a course of prednisolone for an infective exacerbation of COPD. He also gives a history of alcohol excess, drinking 2 litres of cider each day. His diet is poor, and he describes a several-week history of occasional upper abdominal pain prior to his presentation today, though the pain has never been this severe. His abdomen is generally tender and guarded, more so in the epigastric and hypochondriac regions.

What are your differential diagnoses?

Acute pancreatitis, gastritis, peptic ulceration +/- perforation, cholecystitis, cardiac cause such as myocardial ischaemia.

Which investigations would you order and how will they help narrow down your differential?

• Routine biochemistry:
>   o deranged LFTs may suggest biliary cause
>   o amylase 3 x normal is diagnostic for pancreatitis
>   o raised cardiac markers e.g. troponin I suggest an ischaemic cardiac event
• ECG: to rule out myocardial ischaemia
• Imaging: erect chest radiograph +/- CT – pneumoperitoneum is suggestive of perforation. Inflammation and fat stranding on CT in related to gallbladder or pancreas may suggest cholecystitis or pancreatitis respectively.

A CT scan is organised in the Emergency department.

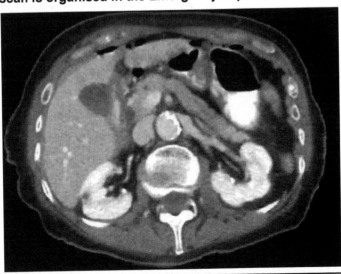

PATHOLOGY

What does the CT scan show?

This is an axial cut CT scan at the level of the stomach and first part of the duodenum. It clearly shows free air within the peritoneal cavity. There is thickening of the antrum of the stomach and first part of the duodenum. These are suggestive of viscus perforation. In the context of the patient scenario above, perforated peptic ulcer seems the likely source.

In some causes a discontinuity in the mucosal wall or a blush of contrast from the GI tract may highlight the exact site of perforation.

How would you manage this patient in the first instance?

The patient should be stabilised following an ABCDE approach with oxygen applied, IV access with two large-bore cannulas and fluid resuscitation and identification and correction of life-threatening haemodynamic abnormalities. The patient should be catheterised to monitor fluid balance and appropriate analgesia should be administered to ensure the patient is comfortable. Escalate as appropriate – this is likely to involve discussion with the registrar and/or consultant as well as informing the relevant theatre and anaesthetic staff. It may also be prudent to alert the ITU team.

What is the definition of an ulcer?

An ulcer is defined as a lesion or breach of the skin or a mucosal membrane. A peptic ulcer is therefore a defect in the gastric or duodenal wall that extends through the muscularis mucosa into the deeper layers of the wall.
• Peptic ulcers are usually chronic, solitary lesions.
• They occur most commonly in the duodenum (80%), followed by the stomach (19%). A small number (approximately 1%) are seen in other sites such as Meckel's diverticulum, oesophagus, or jejunum.

What is the pathophysiology of peptic ulcer disease?

Peptic ulceration is caused by the action of acidic gastric content upon the mucosa of the GI tract. The pathophysiology involves two interlinked processes – an increase in gastric acid secretion as well as a decrease (breach) in the mucosal protective barriers/defences.

What physiological mechanisms are in place to protect against peptic ulceration?

A normal GI tract protects itself from injury by the acidity of gastric contents via several mechanisms, outlined below. An alteration in any one of these factors can predispose to peptic ulceration.
• Mucosal defences:
  o Integrity of the mucosa (maintained by production of prostaglandins, especially PGE2 which has a trophic effect of mucosal cells)
  o Tight cell-cell junction – minimises areas of weakness/possibility for breaches.
  o Luminal cells (in direct contact with gastric contents and enzymes) are more resistant to the acidic environment produced.

• Extra-mucosal defences:
  o Generation of an alkaline environment and favourable pH gradient– bicarbonate secretion from the mucosa leads to a pH on its surface of 7, compared to 2 within the stomach lumen.
  o Mucus Cap – a hydrophobic layer secreted by mucosal cells containing hydrogen carbonate, which buffers the acid.

List the main causes and risk factors of peptic ulceration.

PATHOLOGY

Predisposing factors for peptic ulceration include:
• Increased alcohol intake causes decreased pyloric competence, in turn increasing the volume of acidic gastric contents in the duodenum.
• Smoking (similar mechanism to alcohol).
• Helicobacter pylori infection – see question 9
• Drugs, in particular NSAIDS or corticosteroids – these block the action of cyclo-oxygenase 1 (COX1) enzymes which are involved in the production of gut-mucosa prostaglandins (mainly PGE2). Inhibition of prostaglandin synthesis in the GI tract causes increased gastric acid secretion as well as decreased bicarbonate secretion, decreased mucus secretion and decreased trophic effects on epithelial mucosa.
• Co-morbidities – alcoholic cirrhosis, COPD, hyperparathyroidism and chronic kidney disease are all linked to increased risk of peptic ulceration. This is thought to be related to gastric acid production secondary to hypercalcaemia-driven increased gastrin secretion.
• Genetic – exact mechanisms are unclear. There is a higher incidence of peptic ulceration in certain subgroups, includeing those with HLA – B5, blood group O or type "A" personalities.
• Environmental stress– Cushing's ulceration is seen in patients with severe head injury. Curling's ulcers are seen in patients recovering from burns. Similarly, there is increased incidence in patients following major surgery. This phenomenon may be linked to perturbation of the blood flow to the gastric mucosa.
• Zollinger-Ellison disease – presence of gastrinomas (gastrin-secreting tumours of the pancreatic islet cells) leading to gastric hypersecretion.

What is the likely cause in this case and why is it important to identify?

This patient has several risk factors for peptic ulcer disease – increased alcohol intake, smoking, COPD and recent corticosteroid use. All are possible causes and should be managed on this admission, however the most important to identify quickly in this scenario is the alcoholism. This will require immediate attention. Care must be taken to appropriately treat the patient for alcohol withdrawal using the local hospital protocol (usually chlordiazepoxide and vitamin B12 reducing regime).

What is Helicobacter pylori?

• Gram-negative flagellated micro-aerophillic bacillus
• Specific for human gastric mucosa
• Research suggests up to half the world's population are colonised with this bacterium.
• Is causally linked to the pathogenesis of peptic ulceration through several mechanisms-
    o Produces ammonia (which is directly toxic to mucosal cells)
    o Increases gastrin and subsequently gastric acid production
    o Disrupts the mucosal barrier by adhering to cells and allowing the inward passage of enzymes and acid
    o Stimulates an autoimmune response against the mucosal epithelium.
• Has also been shown to be associated with gastric MALT (mucosa-assosiated lymphoid tissue) lymphoma, gastric cancer and ischaemic heart disease.

What methods are available to test for H.pylori?

There are several possible ways of testing for H.Pylori infection/colonisation. These can be grouped as either non-invasive or invasive.

Non-invasive:
• Carbon-13 urea breath test
    o Good sensitivity and specificity.
    o Urea is labelled with a non-radioactive marker (carbon-13) and ingested

o Urea is split into ammonia and 13-C-labelled CO_2 in the presence of H.pylori.
o This labelled CO_2 can then be detected in the patients' breath samples using mass spectrometry.
- Serology
    o Detects H.pylori antibodies in the blood stream
- Stool testing
    o Stool antigen testing.

Invasive:
- Quick urease test, such as the Campylobacter-like organism (CLO) test
    o Tissue biopsy from the antrum of the stomach tested (biopsy taken endoscopically)
    o Biopsy left in culture medium containing urea and a pH indicator solution
    o Working on the basis that H. pylori produces ammonia in the presence of urea, the solution becomes more alkaline if H. pylori is present
- Histology
    o Biopsies taken at endoscopy are used and examined with stains which detect H. pylori– commonly modified Giemsa stain

Which method can be used to assess eradication of Helicobacter pylori?

- Urease breath test is the only test suitable for repeated use to assess for eradication.
- As antibodies can persist for up to 6-12 months post-treatment, serological tests cannot be used to assess for eradication.
- CLO testing and histology are more invasive, requiring gastroscopy and biopsy, and as such are not appropriate means of repeat testing due to the inherent risks of the procedure.

How would you treat Helicobacter pylori colonisation?

H. Pylori can be eradicated with several treatment protocols. Each trust may have a preferred method, but the underlying principles are the same – the use of a proton-pump inhibitor and two synergistic oral antibiotics. This is known as triple therapy. Two different antibiotics are used to reduce the risk of drug resistance occurring. Treatment occurs over 7-14 days, and this length of treatment can impact on patient compliance. Treatment failure occurs in approximately 20% of cases, with the most common causes being poor compliance and antibiotic resistance. The most frequently used eradication protocol (as recommended by NICE in the UK) is:

- PPI – no specific PPI has been shown to be more effective, as long as equivalent doses are used i.e. 40mg omeprazole is comparable 30mg lansoprazole
- Amoxicillin (1g given three times per day)
- Either clarithromycin (500mg) or metronidazole (400mg) – each three times per day

What are the possible complications of peptic ulcer disease?

There are several potential complications that occur secondary to peptic ulcer disease (see below). Only about half of patients presenting with complicated peptic ulcer disease describe a history of preceding dyspeptic symptoms.
- Perforation
    o Perforation in peptic ulcer disease in more common in the older age groups (but can occur in all ages). In patients over the age of 70, peptic ulcer perforation carries a mortality risk of approximately 20%
    o Classical presentation is that of sudden onset epigastric pain, progressing over hours to peritonitis
    o Approximately 80% of patients will have an identifiable pneumoperitoneum on

PATHOLOGY

erect chest radiograph
- Bleeding
    o Accounts for 70-80% of upper gastrointestinal bleeds
    o Presents as haematemesis, malaena or, less commonly, as haemorrhage per rectum/haematochezia (in briskly bleeding ulcers).
    o Posterior wall duodenal ulcers and gastric ulcers can cause bleeding due to their close proximity to the gastroduodenal and left gastric arteries respectively. However, in most cases the bleeding is caused by the erosion of an artery in the base of the ulcer itself.
    o In approximately 80% of patients, bleeding from a peptic ulcer stops spontaneously, but in the remainder further intervention is required.

The Rockall risk scoring system attempts to identify patients at risk of adverse outcomes following acute upper GI bleeding. It utilises a combination of clinical criteria as well as endoscopic findings. A score of greater than 8 carries a higher risk of mortality, while less than three has the best prognosis.

SUMMARY

Peptic ulcer disease classically presents with burning epigastric pain, often related to eating. Classically, gastric ulcers are more symptomatic after food and duodenal ulcers more symptomatic when fasted. They may present with shock from visceral perforation or haemorrhage. Suspicions should be raised in patients with history of high alcohol intake and NSAID/steroid use. Immediate management should focus on resuscitation and analgesia with treatment of the underlying causes. This is largely medical, including PPIs and H. pylori eradication. Surgery tends to be reserved for the emergency setting or the treatment of complications

TOP TIPS

➕ Remember during clerking to explore possible causes of peptic ulceration. This will help to guide further management. Alcohol is an important risk factor/cause of peptic ulceration to consider – this needs immediate treatment as alcohol withdrawal can have serious sequelae.

➕ Remember to look out for the possible complications associated with peptic ulceration. It is important not to miss these, as bleeding or visceral perforation may be life threatening.

2.6 | Blunt Trauma

Scenario

A 19-year-old female with no significant past medical history is involved in a road traffic accident. She is the restrained front seat passenger in a head on collision with another car at 40 miles per hour. She is taken to her nearest major trauma centre. On primary survey she is found to be hypotensive and tachycardic with a GCS of 14. There is tenderness and surgical emphysema on palpation over the left sided thoracic wall. On abdominal examination there was noted to be generalised abdominal tenderness, maximally on the left side, with associated distension and bruising over the left upper quadrant and flank. Urine analysis confirmed beta HCG was negative but was suggestive for trace protein and blood.

How would you manage this patient in the first instance?

The patient should be managed according to the ATLS protocol. The patient should be assessed and stabilised by a trauma team, following the ATLS ABCDE approach whilst simultaneously securing access with 2 x wide bore IV cannulas, initiating fluid resuscitation as appropriate and correction of any identified life-threatening abnormalities. Routine bloods, including FBC, clotting screen, U+Es and group and save should be collected. The initial assessment is the primary survey, which aims to quickly identify and correct any imminently life-threatening problems. Once a patient is stable, the secondary survey assesses the patient in fine detail, including musculoskeletal and neurological systems, for possible injuries. This survey helps guide further imaging and longer-term management plans.

The ATLS approach to the ABCDE algorithm is as follows:
• Airway maintenance with cervical spine protection
• Breathing and ventilation
• Circulation with hemorrhage control
• Disability (neurological status)
• Exposure and environmental control (completely undress and assess the patient whilst avoiding hypothermia and maintaining dignity)

What are the key aspects of history required for assessment of trauma patients and how can they be obtained?

During the assessment (often at the time of the secondary survey) a brief history is elicited. It is important to gather as much information regarding the traumatic event itself (since certain mechanisms of injury are associated with specific patterns of injury and may help focus further assessment). It is also vital to know pertinent past medical history and current medications. The mnemonic AMPLE is often used:
• Allergies
• Medications
• Past medical history
• Last ate/ last menstrual period in females of child bearing age
• Event/environment related to the injury

In the event that the patient is unconscious or unable to provide a history, other sources need to be considered. These can be collateral history from family or friends, old clinical notes within the hospital or information on the patient itself (e.g ID/allergy bracelet)

Given the primary survey, what injuries do you suspect?

Examination findings include:

PATHOLOGY

• GCS 14 – possible head injury

• Surgical emphysema over left sided chest wall – suggestive of left pneumothorax. The associated left chest wall tenderness may suggest underlying rib fractures which may have caused the pneumothorax. Haemopneumothorax should be considered.

• Left sided abdominal bruising – may be simple musculoskeletal injury but need to rule out underlying visceral injury – bruising in this area requires assessment for splenic/left kidney injury.

• Hypotension and tachycardia – suggestive of shock. In a polytrauma setting such as this, with other significant abdominal signs (bruising, distension, tenderness) and no other obvious source of bleeding, a shocked patient should be managed for presumed intra-abdominal/pelvic bleeding until proven otherwise.

What investigations are required?

Simultaneously to IV access being gained, routine bloods should be collected and sent. In this context this should include FBC, U+Es, venous blood gas, clotting screen and group and save (or cross match if active bleeding is suspected)

Following a primary survey, basic trauma films are obtained – this specifically focuses on the chest and pelvis – it helps further assess for life threatening injuries that may not have been picked up – e.g. pneumo/haemothorax, or pelvic fractures.

If the patient is stable enough, most would undergo a full trauma CT series (head through to pelvis, including C-Spine), which aims to assess and characterise all injuries present.

Please interpret this plain chest radiograph

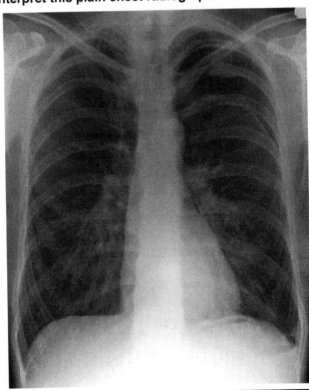

This is a plain chest radiograph. It demonstrates a left sided pneumothorax which associated left rib fractures to ribs 3-5 and some surgical emphysema to the adjacent soft tissue. The trachea is not shifted from midline, suggesting that this is not a tension pneumothorax. There is no evidence of effusion suggestive of haemothorax. A pneumothorax can be identified on CXR by visible visceral pleural edge seen as a very thin, sharp white line and no lung markings are seen peripheral to this line.

What would be the significance of a 1st rib fracture in this context?

A first rib fracture can be considered a hallmark of severe trauma. They are rare and imply a significant force related to the mechanism of injury. If a first rib fracture is identified, further assessment for other potential injuries should be carried out. In particular, injuries to adjacent structures such as the cervical spine, subclavian vessels and brachial plexus. The force required to fracture a first rib should also alert the trauma team to the possibility of massive generalised injury.

How would you manage this pneumothorax? How would the management differ if this were a tension pneumothorax?

This pneumothorax would need to be managed with an intercostal chest drain. The negative pressure created by the chest drain system helps to remove any air or fluid from the space.
The procedure is as follows:
• Use of aseptic technique and personal protective equiptment
• Site = mid-axillary line, fifth intercostal space (on expiration, the diaphragm reaches the 5th intercostal space therefore no drain should be placeddlower than this level). Similarly, the use of the "triangle of safety" is a safe guide for placement. This is a triangle created by: Mid-axillary line, lateral boarder of pectoralis major and the imaginary horizontal line from the nipple.
•An incision is made along the upper border of the rib below the intercostal space to be used. The drain tract will be directed over the top of the lower rib to avoid the intercostal vessels (lying below each rib).
• Use blunt dissection to reach the pleura (using finger, Robert's forceps etc)
• Puncture the pleura with scissors or forceps. If you are using a large bore tube, you may need to insert a finger to remove any adherent lung
• A large-bore (e.g. 32 French) chest tube is mounted on the clamp and passed along the tract into the pleural cavity.
• The tube is connected to an underwater seal and sutured / secured in place.
• The chest is re-examined to confirm effect (equal expansion, air entry throughout, reduced respiratory rate, improved saturations) and another chest X-ray is taken to confirm placement & position.
• Analysis of the drain output is an important part of the assessment. If it is blood, high-volume or arterial blood are much more likely to require further intervention (e.g. thoracotomy). Drainage of intestinal contents implies either an oesophageal injury or stomach /bowel injury with associated diaphragmatic tear, while a persistent air leak implies an underlying lung laceration.
If the pneumothorax was a tension pneumothorax, the management would differ in that emergency needle thoracocentesis would first be performed, by inserting a large-bore cannula into the second intercostals space in the mid-clavicular line.

What is significance of the urinalysis findings in this context

The urinalysis demonstrates the presence of non-visible haematuria. Any post-traumatic haematuria should alert clinicians to the risk of renal tract injury. In blunt trauma such as this, non-visible haematuria warrants careful clinical assessment. If the patient is symp-

PATHOLOGY

tomatic (e.g. flank pain or bruising/ other abdominal symptoms) then imaging such as contrast CT is appropriate. Asymptomatic patients with non-visible haematuria following blunt trauma may just need repeat urinalysis in 1-2 weeks to ensure resolution.

The presence of visible haematuria is much more suggestive of a significant injury somewhere along the renal tract (including the prostate in males). All cases of visible haematuria in the context of trauma need to be investigated. Cases related to abdominal/pelvic penetrating injury are likely to need surgical exploration.

In female patients, knowing pregnancy status is important. Pregnancy can present a source of concealed bleeding in a patient with abdominal trauma. It may also influence investigation/intervention, and warrant input from obstetric teams.

What other clinical findings may raise suspicions of significant abdominal injury?

- Complaints of abdominal pain
- Abdominal tenderness on palpation
- Peritonism
- Abdominal distension
- Bruising
  - o Seatbelt sign – bruising in position of seat belt in restrained passengers/drivers may suggest underlying visceral injury. Bowel and mesentery are particularly at risk via this mechanism
  - o Grey Turner's sign – bruising in the flanks. It is suggestive of bleeding in the retroperitoneum
  - o Cullen's sign – bruising in the subcutaneous tissue around the umbilicus. It is suggestive of intra-abdominal bleeding (bleeding and oedema tracks up towards the umbilicus along the falciform ligament)
- Haematuria/blood at the urethral meatus
- Haemodynamic instability with no other obvious source of bleeding
- Other injuries may raise suspicions of abdominal injuries – lower rib fractures may be associated with liver, renal or splenic laceration. Pelvis fractures may cause bowel, bladder and rectal injuries, or disrupt the pelvic venous plexus.

A CT trauma series is requested as part of the patients' initial assessment. A slice from the CT abdomen and pelvis is shown below. Discuss the findings.

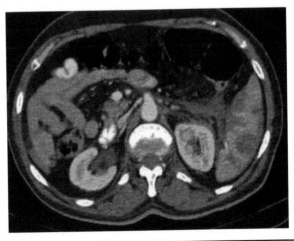

There is a grade II splenic injury and grade III left renal injury. There is also free fluid (presumably blood) seen, with perinephric and peri-splenic haematoma.

Describe how splenic and renal injuries are graded

Splenic Grading

Grade I	Grade II	Grade III	Grade IV	Grade V
capsular laceration <1 cm depth	laceration 1-3 cm depth	laceration >3 cm depth or involving vessels	laceration involving segmental or hilar vessels with major devascularisation (>25% of spleen)	hilar vascular injury with devascularised spleen
subcapsular haematoma <10% of surface area	subcapsular haematoma 10-50% of surface area	subcapsular haematoma >50% of surface area or expanding		Shattered spleen
	intraparenchymal haematoma <5cm in diameter	intraparenchymal haematoma >5cm or expanding		

Renal Grading

Grade I	Grade II	Grade III	Grade IV	Grade V
Contusion, no laceration	superficial laceration <1cm depth, not involving the collecting system	superficial laceration >1cm depth, not involving the collecting system	laceration extends to renal pelvis, or there is evidence of urinary extravasation	Shattered kidney
			vascular: injury to main renal artery or vein with contained haemorrhage	complete laceration or thrombus of the main renal artery or vein
			segmental infarctions without associated lacerations	avulsion of renal hilum, devascularisation of a kidney due to hilar injury
			expanding subcapsular haematomas compressing the kidney	

With this particular modality, it would be difficult to rule out a renal injury greater than grade III. A renal excretory phase CT would clarify if there was a collecting system injury/ urine extravasation suggesting grade IV injury or greater.

PATHOLOGY

How would you manage this patients' abdominal injuries?

This patient has a grade II splenic injury and a grade III left renal injury. There was evidence of free blood in the abdomen, which may suggest active bleeding (though it is difficult to comment on this with certainty based on this slice alone, as there was no evidence of contrast blush to imply extravasation). The patient is also hypotensive and tachycardic. This is suggestive of haemodynamic instability warranting immediate intervention – this may be in the form of surgical exploration (e.g. splenectomy) or interventional radiology (embolisation of the bleeding vessel).

Not all low-grade solid organ injuries (grades I-III, many grade IV injuries) require surgery. A stable patient may be managed conservatively, with observation and serial examination. Facilities for surgery/interventional radiology should be available should the patient deteriorate.

What issue needs to be considered post-operatively following a splenectomy?

Post splenectomy, a patient is at risk of infection from encapsulated bacteria, in particular Streptococcus pneumoniae, Haemophilus influenzae and Neisseria meningitidis. Post-splenectomy sepsis occurs in approximately 5% of patients without the appropriate precautions:

• Vaccination against pneumoccocus and Hib- 14 days post surgery.
• Lifelong prophylactic oral antibiotics – phenoxymethylpenicillin or macrolides are recommended.

SUMMARY

Management of trauma patients requires a thorough systematic approach utilising the ATLS protocol of primary followed by secondary survey. The aim of this approach is to ensure significant and potentially life-threatening injuries are identified and managed quickly. Blunt abdominal trauma is commonly associated with solid organ injury (e.g. liver, spleen, kidney), as was the case in this scenario. The management of these sorts of injuries is often supportive. However, peritonism, unexplained hypotension and ongoing bleeding may require emergency surgical exploration.

TOP TIPS

✚ A brief history *(including collateral history)* is an important part of the assessment of trauma. Understanding a patient's co-morbidities and drug history allows for a more thorough examination. For example, patients with cardiac disease or taking beta-blockers may not mount the same physiological response to trauma and can have falsely reassuring observations.

✚ Remember that certain mechanisms of injuries are associated with certain patterns of injury and this may help focus assessment and management.

PATHOLOGY

2.7 Liver Disease

Scenario

A middle aged man with a history of alcoholism presents to the emergency department with complaints of abdominal distension. On examination he is found to be hypotensive with a bounding pulse, while general inspection reveals icteric sclera, gynaecomastia and dilated tortuous veins over the abdominal wall itself. Abdominal examination confirms that he is indeed very distended and that this is generally quite tender and tense. There is noted to be shifting dullness on abdominal wall percussion.

From the examination findings, what is your differential diagnosis?

The main differential diagnosis should be of chronic liver disease with associated ascites and portal hypertension. From the history of alcoholism and the examination findings, the likely cause is cirrhosis. Other potential differentials include abdominal mass (either malignant or benign, primary or secondary - possibly hepatic or perihepatic in view of other clinical signs) or bowel obstruction.

How should you manage this patient in the first instance?

The patient should be managed according to the ABCDE protocol, with efficient identification and correction of any significant abnormalities in physiological parameters. IV access should be gained and routine bloods collected. When the patient is stable, a more thorough clinical history and examination may be conducted. These should focus on eliciting the severity of the liver disease plus any associated complications, as well as identifying potential underlying causes (if unknown). Investigations should complement the clinical assessment:

- **Bloods:**
  - o Liver function tests (to assess severity of disease)
  - o Clotting studies (to assess severity of disease)
  - o Metabolic screen – e.g. serum copper, iron studies (possible causes)
  - o Hepatitis screen – A, B, C, D, E, plus EBV/CMV (possible causes)
  - o Autoimmune screen – anti-mitochondrial antibodies associated with primary biliary cirrhosis, anti-smooth-muscle antibodies associated with autoimmune hepatitis
- **Imaging:**
  - o Ultrasound scan or CT scan may characterise the type of cirrhosis, identify hepatic or biliary duct dilatation or extrinsic obstructive causes, and help to record disease evolution (with serial investigations).

What other clinical signs might you associate with liver disease and cirrhosis?

In the case above, you can pick out many clinical signs associated with liver disease and cirrhosis – including jaundice, gynaecomastia, ascites and caput medusae (engorged superficial epigastric veins secondary to portal hypertension). Other signs related to liver disease may include:
- Palpable liver edge
- Excoriation - secondary to icteric pruritus
- Stigmata of chronic liver disease
  - o Fingernail clubbing

PATHOLOGY

o Leukonychia - white spots on fingernails, suggestive of hypoalbuminaemia
o Palmar erythema
o Dupuytren's contracture – tethering along the flexor tendons of the fingers
o Spider naevi – more than 5 is suggestive of liver disease. Seen in distribution of superior vena cava. They are caused by high circulating oestrogen levels as a cirrhotic liver is unable to break down oestrogen.
o Loss of body hair, testicular atrophy – caused by high levels of circulating oestrogen
o Asterixis/liver flap
• Portal hypertension
  o Splenomegaly
  o Right heart failure
• Xanthomata - seen in biliary cirrhosis
• Kayser-Fleischer rings – cooper coloured rings in the iris, associated with Wilson's disease
• Bronzed complexion – seen in haemochromatosis

Discuss the possible causes of cirrhosis

In the UK, Cirrhosis is the most common cause of liver failure and alcohol is the most common cause of cirrhosis. Other causes include:
• Congenital
  o Haemochromatosis
  o Alpha-1-anti-trypsin deficiency
  o Wilson's disease
• Acquired
  o Toxins – drug-induced (e.g. amiodarone, methotrexate)
  o Infection
  o Hepatitis B
  o Hepatitis C
  o Schistosomiasis - common in the tropics, causes fibrosis and portal hyperten sion (technically not a true cirrhosis)
• Autoimmune
  o Primary biliary cirrhosis
  o Primary sclerosing cholangitis
  o Chronic autoimmune hepatitis
  o Secondary biliary cirrhosis, caused by gallstones, biliary strictures, cholangitis
  o Sarcoidosis

Describe the pathological features of cirrhosis?

While the clinical picture and imaging (US and CT) may point towards a diagnosis of cirrhosis, a true diagnosis cannot be made without a biopsy. Histologically, cirrhosis is characterised by loss of the normal histological architecture secondary to fibrosis of the liver parenchyma, nodular regeneration and hepatocellular necrosis. Three forms of this pattern exist:
• Micronodular – uniform nodules <4mm in size, separated by thin fibrous septa
• Macronodular – larger nodules, irregularly distributed throughout the liver
• Mixed pattern

What are the main complications of cirrhosis? What impact does it have on a patients' fitness for surgery?

The main complications associated with cirrhosis are liver failure, hepatocellular carcinoma, portal hypertension, ascites and deterioration following surgery.

PATHOLOGY

Cirrhosis creates an environment of hyperdynamic circulation with increased cardiac output and decreased systemic vascular resistance (with increased resistance in the portal system). Perfusion of the cirrhotic liver is decreased- portal blood flow is reduced as a result of portal hypertension, and arterial blood flow decreased because of impaired autoregulation. Surgery can exacerbate this state and precipitate hepatic decompensation with resultant encephalopathy, ascites, renal failure and haemorrhage. Factors contributing to decreased hepatic blood flow intraoperatively include hypotension, hemorrhage and vasoactive anaesthetic drugs.

What is portal hypertension?

The term portal hypertension refers to abnormally high pressure within the portal venous system. It is defined as a portal pressure of greater than 12mmHg (normal range 5-20mmHg). Increased vascular resistance (secondary to factors such as mechanical constriction on the portal system from fibrosis) and increased portal blood flow (secondary to increased cardiac output, hypervolaemia and arterial hypotension) are important factors in the development of portal hypertension.

List the possible causes of portal hypertension

Causes of portal hypertension can be classified according to their location in relation to the liver and associated vasculature.
• Pre-hepatic
> o Portal vein thrombosis
> o Congenital portal vein atresia
> o Phlebitis of the portal vein from intra-abdominal infection
> o Thrombosed porto-caval shunt

• Hepatic
> o Cirrhosis – the most common cause, with alcoholic cirrhosis being the most abundant form in the UK
> o Schistosomiasis infection
> o Chronic active hepatitis – infective, autoimmune, drug-induced
> o Multiple hepatic metastases

• Post-hepatic
> o Budd-Chiari syndrome (thrombosis of hepatic vein)
> o Constrictive pericarditis
> o Right heart failure
> o Tricuspid valve incompetence
> o Pulmonary hypertension

What is the management of portal hypertension?

Portal hypertension in its own right is difficult to treat effectively. The most effective means is by treating the underlying cause and liver transplantation, though this is not possible in all cases. Management may also focus on the treatment of the complications of portal hypertension, rather that the hypertension itself.

Medical management:
• Beta-blockers such as propanolol can reduce portal pressure and reduce rate of bleeding in patients with varices. Recent evidence suggests beta-blockers may also protect against spontaneous bacterial peritonitis in cases of ascites. The mechanism of this is somewhat unclear but may be through increasing gastrointestinal motility and transit.
• Nitrates – may reduce portal hypertension. Often used in conjunction with beta-blockers.
• Anticoagulation in Budd-Chiari syndrome
• Terlipressin and octreotide is used in management of oesophageal variceal bleeding by reducing variceal pressure.
Invasive/surgical management:

PATHOLOGY

• TIPS - Transjugular intrahepatic portosystemic shunt. A stent is placed radiologically to create a shunt from the portal system to the hepatic system. This decompresses the portal system, reducing the pressure within it.
• Porta-caval shunt – decompresses the portal system via the vena cava
• Liver transplantation
• Endoscopic ligation or scleropathy for varices

What are the possible complications of portal hypertension?

The four most important complications of portal hypertension are the development of ascites, splenomegaly, liver failure and varices

What are varices? Where may varices develop and why?

Varices are engorged, dilated veins. Raised portal pressures divert blood from the congested portal system through collaterals connecting to the systemic veins. There are a number of sites of portosystemic anastomoses:
• Between the left gastric vein (portal) and oesophageal branches of the azygos vein (systemic)
• Between the superior (portal) and inferior rectal veins (systemic)
• Between the obliterated umbilical vein (portal) and the superior/inferior epigastric veins (systemic)
• Retroperitoneal anastomoses

How does ascites develop?

Ascites is the accumulation of fluid within the abdomen. Its pathophysiology is multifactorial. The basic underlying principle is extravasation of fluid from plasma to peritoneal fluid. Various factors play a role:
• Portal hypertension (increased hydrostatic pressure)
• Sodium and water retention in the intra-vascular compartment secondary to increased aldosterone activity
• Low serum albumin (decreased intravascular osmotic pressure)
• Increased pressure within the hepatic lymphatic system can also result in lymph transudation from liver.

List the possible causes of ascites

Causes of ascites can be classified by whether they produce a transudate or exudate collection. The distinction between a transudate and an exudate is made according to the serum-ascites albumin gradient (SAAG). A figure >11g/L (high SAAG) implies it is a transudate, while <11g/L (low SAAG) is an exudate.
Causes of transudate ascites
• Hepatic failure
• Cirrhosis
• Hepatic venous occlusion
• Liver metastasis
• Cardiac failure
• Constrictive pericarditis
• Kwashiorkor

Causes of exudate ascites
• Other malignancy
• Pancreatitis
• Nephrotic syndrome
• Infection – bacterial, peritoneal TB, fungal
• Bowel pathology – obstruction, infarction

What is the management for ascites?

Medical management:
• Low-salt diet and fluid restriction
• Diuretics – potassium sparing such as spironolactone
• Medical management as per portal hypertension

Invasive/surgical management:
• Paracentesis is indicated in diuretic-resistant ascites, or if the ascites becomes tense or infected
• Peritoneal venous shunting. This involves the creation of a shunt between peritoneal cavity and internal jugular vein, tunnelled in the subcutaneous tissue.
• TIPS/porto-caval shunt, as in management of portal hypertension

What are the possible complications of ascites?

• Spontaneous bacterial peritonitis.
  o 10-30% incidence
  o Mortality risk of 20%
  o Most commonly involve E.coli, streptococci, enterococci
  o Diagnosed if ascitic fluid contains >250/mm3 neutrophils
  o Empirical antibiotics – as per hospital guidelines – often third generation cephelosporins
• Hepatorenal syndrome
  o Is the development of renal failure in a patient with advanced liver disease
  o A complication of cirrhosis with ascites
  o Thought to be due to the presence of nephrotoxins normally eliminated by the liver, plus circulatory changes (decreased systemic vascular resistance, low systemic arterial pressure, intra-renal vasoconstriction) resulting in hypoperfusion of the kidneys
• Hepatic hydrothorax
  o Defined as a transudate pleural effusion, usually greater than 500 mL, in patients with portal hypertension and ascites, without any other underlying primary cardiopulmonary cause.
  o Treatment involves reduction of portal hypertension if possible, pleurodesis, diuretics
  o A chest drain is not indicated unless there is an empyema to be drained as can precipitate hepato-renal syndrome and electrolyte imbalance. In addition, the collection often recurs as soon as the drain is removed.

SUMMARY

Chronic liver disease and cirrhosis is associated with a classic collection of clinical signs, including jaundice, spider naevi, caput medusa, asterixis and gynaecomastia. Portal hypertension often arises within the context of cirrhosis. Perhaps the most important complication of portal hypertension is the development of varices. Though these can develop in a number of anatomical sites, oesophageal varices are the most likely to bleed. Haemorrhage from bleeding oesophageal varices is often severe and may be life-threatening. Management of these patients' should focus on rapid fluid resuscitation and arrest of bleeding, usually via endoscopic banding or injection.

PATHOLOGY

TOP TIPS

➕ Clinical history and examination is vital to establish the likely cause of portal hypertension and liver disease, which should guide treatment in most cases. Remember it is very important in particular to identify alcoholism, as alcohol withdrawal has serious sequelae and will need to be managed in the acute setting.

➕ Portal hypertension is likely to present as one of its complications – ascites, liver failure or variceal bleeding.

➕ Causes of ascites – transudate vs. exudate – is a common exam question.

PATHOLOGY

2.8 | Peripheral Vasuclar Disease

Scenario

An 80-year-old man presents on the advice of his general practitioner complaining of persistent pain in his left leg for three days, which has become intolerable over the last 12 hours. It is now associated with a numb feeling in the foot. The patient is taking medication for hypertension, hypercholesterolemia, type two diabetes and atrial fibrillation (though he is not anticoagulated due to a high risk of falls). He has a history of myocardial infarction 5 years prior, prostatic malignancy and lower back pain. He is a current smoker of 20 cigarettes a day. On examination, his left leg looks pale and feels cold distal to the knee in comparison to the right. On the same side, there is also noted to be venous guttering. Sensation seemed slightly reduced over the left foot itself. Weak femoral pulses are palpable bilaterally, with no pedal pulses distally on either leg. The referring GP was unable to measure an ABPI.

What is your differential diagnosis?

Acute limb ischaemia, compartment syndrome, neurogenic cause/spinal stenosis

How would you manage this man in the first instance?

The patient needs to be admitted to hospital for further assessment and intervention. They should be managed according to the ABCDE protocol, with efficient identification and correction of any significant abnormalities in physiological parameters. IV access should be gained and routine bloods collected.

When the patient is stable and appropriate analgesia has been administered, a more thorough clinical history and examination may be conducted. This should focus on eliciting the extent of ischaemia and considering possible causes. This can influence management. Signs such as paraesthesia, paralysis and fixed mottling of the skin are late signs and often reflect irreversible ischaemic damage not suitable for revascularisation. A history of intermittent claudication suggests preceding peripheral arterial disease. Is atrial fibrillation or a popliteal aneurysm present suggesting possible embolic aetiology? Intravenous heparin should be commenced while definitive management is being planned.

What investigations will be helpful in this case?

Investigations should complement the clinical assessment:
- Bloods:
    - o Baseline full blood count - ischaemia is exacerbated by anaemia.
    - o Baseline renal function – heparin and CT contrast are nephrotoxic. If the limb is revascularised, this can precipitate reperfusion injury to the kidney.
    - o Clotting studies - to help guide anticoagulation treatment.
    - o Thrombophilia screen – may identify coagulopathy as possible cause.
- ECG and echocardiogram – to identify arrhythmia as a possible source of emboli.
- Imaging:
    - o Ultrasound scan (duplex) or CT angiogram,
- Aortic ultrasound – identify aneurysm, a possible source of emboli.
- Arterial duplex to assess patency of arterial tree and blood flow.
- Venous duplex – used to map suitable vessels for vein harvesting in possible bypass grafting.
- CT – helps identify exact location of arterial occlusion, helpful in treatment planning.

PATHOLOGY

What is meant by the term 'ABPI'?

The ankle-brachial pressure index (or ABPI) is the ratio of the pressure at the ankle, compared to the brachial artery. It is a quick, non-invasive, reproducible means of assessing lower limb arterial flow. It can be used to help quantify the severity of present peripheral arterial disease, but is more helpful in assessing change in disease over time (i.e. before versus after intervention).

An ABPI measurement of 1 is normal. Values of 0.9-0.5 implies the presence of peripheral arterial disease and intermittent claudication is likely to be present in this range. Measurements of 0.5-0.3 are likely to correlate with rest pain and an ABPI <0.2 is associated with tissue loss (ulceration/gangrene).

An ABPI less than 0.90 has been shown to have a sensitivity of 90% and a specificity of 98% for detecting a lower-extremity stenosis of greater than 50%.

Several caveats need to be considered when using ABPI readings clinically. Heavily calcified vessels, as in diabetes or renal disease, are difficult to compress at the ankle and so will give unreliable high readings (usually >1.3). Arterial occlusive disease of the subclavian/axillary vessels bilaterally will also produce unrealistically high readings. Similarly, a patient with particularly high or low systemic blood pressure (brachial reading) can produce inaccurate measurements.

Define critical limb ischaemia?

Critical limb ischaemia is an advanced stage of peripheral arterial disease. It is defined as the presence of rest pain and tissue loss (i.e. arterial ulcers, gangrene) with proven arterial occlusive disease of the affected limb. There is usually an ABPI reading of <0.5.

Define acute limb ischaemia?

Acute limb ischemia is defined as a sudden decrease in limb perfusion that causes a potential threat to limb viability. It classically presents clinically with the "6 P's" :

• Pain
• Pallor
• Pulselessness
• Perishingly cold
• Paraethesia
• Paralysis

Paraesthesia and paralysis are late signs. They imply a degree of irreversible tissue damage.

What is the main cause of peripheral artery disease and critical limb ischaemia?

The underlying pathophysiology of peripheral arterial disease is usually atherosclerosis causing arterial stenosis. This leads to reduced distal blood flow and therefore diminished tissue perfusion. Risk factors for peripheral vascular disease therefore include smoking, hypercholesterolemia, hypertension and diabetes mellitus.

Describe the pathological features of atherosclerosis

Atherosclerosis is a generalised disease which most commonly affects the coronary, cerebral and peripheral vasculature. It tends to affect areas where vessels branch or have areas of irregularity, since these areas generate more turbulent blood flow. The pathological basis of atherosclerosis is multifactorial, involving a process of lipid accumulation, cell migration and inflammation:

• Lipid accumulation in subendothelial macrophages
• Release of intracellular components from cellular necrosis

- Chronic inflammatory environment
- Chronic calcification in vessel wall
- Thickening of tunica intima (caused by smooth muscle hyperplasia)

What aspects of the clinical assessment above suggest that this patient may have a preceding history of peripheral arterial disease?

There are various clues in the case scenario that suggest preceding disease. Firstly, the patient has numerous risk factors for atherosclerosis (smoking, diabetes, hypercholesterolemia, hypertension) and has had an MI in the past which should raise suspicions for peripheral arterial disease. The insidious onset over the last few days implies the presence of a collateral blood supply. Collaterals develop over time to compensate for impaired arterial flow to the limb. In patients with no history of peripheral arterial disease, the sudden occlusion of an artery with no adjacent collateral system would cause very rapid onset (over hours) of the "6 P's" instead. Lastly, there are no palpable pedal pulses on either side – including the currently asymptomatic right leg. This implies the presence of contralateral arterial stenosis as well.

What are the main causes of acute limb ischaemia? What do you think caused this patients symptoms?

Acute limb ischaemia manifests as a result of acute thrombi, emboli, or less commonly trauma. It is difficult to classify the definite cause in this case, since the patient has a number of risk factors for both thrombus (a number of various cardiovascular risk factors, likely atherosclerosis given history of peripheral and cardiac arterial disease) and embolus (atrial fibrillation, malignancy). The two pathophysiologies can often overlap, with an acute embolus lodging at a site of significant atherosclerotic narrowing.

What is difference between an embolus and a thrombus?

An embolus is defined as a mass (such as a thrombus fragment or air bubble) that travels in the bloodstream and lodges in a blood vessel, causing an occlusion. Thrombus is a solid mass of platelets and fibrin that forms locally within a vessel when the clotting mechanism is activated, at the site of an ulcerated atherosclerotic plaque or endothelial cell injury.

What are the management options for a peripheral arterial disease and intermittent claudication?

- Conservative – focuses on cardiovascular risk factor modification. Includes lifestyle advice such as low fat diet, smoking cessation and weight loss. Regular walking is also encouraged to promote the development of collateral blood vessels in the lower limb and help to reduce ischaemic symptoms.
- Medical – NICE recommends "best medical therapy" for patients with claudication. This approach also centres on modification of cardiovascular risk factors. All patients should be prescribed a statin, aspirin and an antihypertensive agent. Good glycaemic control is another essential part of the protocol. Naftidrofuryl oxalate, a vasodilator, may also be prescribed should other methods fail.
- Surgical – typically reserved for those with severe disease or in those whom non-surgical treatment has failed.
    - Angioplasty and stenting – balloon dilatation of a stenosed vessel via percutaneous catheter. Stents may also be placed to keep a vessel lumen patent.
    - Open surgery e.g. bypass graft – the placement of a graft (vein or synthetic PTFE – vein is preferable) across an obstruction.

PATHOLOGY

What are the management options for critical limb ischaemia?

In critical ischaemia, surgical intervention is indicated as the first-line option. Revascularisation options are as listed above – endovascularly or by open surgery. Post-operatively, lifestyle and pharmacological modification of cardiovascular risk factors is extremely important to reduce the risk of future complications and recurrence of stenosis.

What are the management options for acute limb ischaemia?

This is a surgical emergency and immediate admission and intervention is required in order to preserve the limb.
• Anticoagulation – usually an unfractionated heparin infusion, though sometimes low molecule weight heparin or oral anticoagulants are used. Anticoagulation as a definitive treatment tends to only be used in patients who would not be fit for more invasive intervention.
• Embolectomy – emboli can be removed from the arterial lumen via insertion of a fogarty catheter (inserted after open arterial exposure and formation or arterotomy). Open embolectomy is now more rarely performed but remains a management option.
• Bypass graft.

Duration of symptoms is an important consideration in treatment planning. It should be remembered that sensory deficit, such as light touch, two-point tactile discrimination, proprioception, and vibratory perception develop early on. Profound paralysis with complete loss of sensation indicates extensive tissue damage and an irreversible state of ischemia. In this case, primary amputation of the affected limb is likely to be the best intervention, with regard to both patient survival and function/rehabilitation in the future.
In cases of emboli, the source should be identified and treated to reduce risk of recurrent episode. This includes ultrasound duplex to assess for abdominal or popliteal aneurysm, ECG/echocardiogram for cardiac causes etc.

What complications can arise after treatment for acute limb ischaemia?

• Reperfusion injury:
    o Cardiac arrhythmia and acute tubular necrosis secondary to systemic release of blood from the previously ischaemic region – this is high in lactate and potassium.
    o Compartment syndrome due to increased capillary permeability and oedema occurring on reperfusion. The key to management is prevention through prompt revascularisation and a low threshold for fasciotomy.
• Chronic pain syndrome
    o Peripheral nerve damage can occur after periods of acute ischaemia
    o If recognised promptly, can be managed with neuropathic analgesic agents.

SUMMARY

Peripheral arterial disease can present as intermittent claudication (intermittent, reproducible leg pain associated with exertion), critical ischaemia (presence of rest pain and/or tissue loss secondary to significant reduction of tissue) or acute limb ischaemia (sudden complete occlusion of a portion of the arterial tree resulting in pain and eventually irreversible tissue injury). Acute limb ischaemia classically presents with the "6 P's" – pain, pulselessness, perishingly cold, pallor, paraesthesia and paralysis. It is usually caused by a thrombus or embolus. Treatment aims to restore perfusion to the limb. Revascularisation may be via anticoagulation, embolectomy, bypass or endovascular angioplasty or stenting. Extensive tissue loss may warrant amputation.

PATHOLOGY

TOP TIPS

➕ When dealing with acute limb ischaemia, remember the *"6 P's"*. However, do not rely on all 6 being present to make a diagnosis – paraesthesia and paralysis are late signs and suggest irreversible tissue damage.

➕ Patients with preceding peripheral arterial disease may not present in the classical rapid-onset *"6 P's"* of acute limb ischaemia due to the formation of collateral vessels. Instead, their symptoms may have a more protracted onset, or they may present simply with worsening of their chronic symptoms.

➕ Learn the difference in definition and presentation of chronic peripheral arterial disease, critical limb ischaemia and acute limb ischaemia. While restoration of arterial flow is the aim of treatment in all three cases, the specific approaches to management differ between them.

PATHOLOGY

2.9 Abdominal Aortic Aneurysm

Scenario

At 07:00 a man is brought in to hospital by ambulance, following a collapse at home. He complains of severe abdominal pain radiating to his back and left loin and groin, associated with one episode of visible haematuria. He is normotensive but tachycardic. There is abdominal distension and tenderness on palpation centrally and in the left iliac fossa of the abdomen.

The patient is 69 years old with a background of hypertension, hypercholesteraemia and osteoarthritis. He is independent, lives with his wife, smokes 30 cigarettes per day but drinks no alcohol.

What are your main differential diagnoses?

Ruptured abdominal aortic aneurysm (AAA), renal calculi, pyelonephritis, visceral perforation.

This a common exam scenario. In this age group, especially those with cardiovascular risk factors, a ruptured AAA needs to be ruled out before any other diagnosis is made.

How would you manage this patient in the first instance?

The patient should be stabilised following an ABCDE approach with oxygen applied, IV access with two large-bore cannulas, and fluid resuscitation titred to response. Life-threatening haemodynamic abnormalities should be identified and corrected. Routine bloods, including full blood count, renal function, clotting and cross match should be collected. The patient should be catheterised to monitor fluid balance and appropriate analgesia should be administered to ensure the patient is comfortable. Escalate as appropriate – this is likely to involve discussing with your consultant as well as informing the relevant theatre, anaesthetic +/- ITU staff. It is likely this patient will need a CT scan to confirm the suspected diagnosis of AAA, however they will need to stable enough before transfer to the radiology department.

It is important not to underestimate the potential for sudden deterioration in bleeding patients. Tachypnoea and tachycardia may be the only abnormalities at first. Hypotension is a late sign, corresponding to an estimated blood loss of 1500-2000mls

Also, it is important to consider the role of permissive hypotension in patients you suspect are bleeding. This concept involves careful fluid resuscitation to maintain adequate perfusion, but not to raise blood pressure so high as to drive further haemorrhage.

What investigations would you order and how will they help narrow down your differential?

- Routine bloods:
i. FBC – is there a low Hb to suggest bleeding? Or a raised WCC to suggest infection? In the acute setting, a normal haemoglobin can be falsely rassuring- a normal haemoglobin concentration does not preclude acute bleeding.
ii. Renal function – guides intervention in patients with renal calculi and is important to know in patients proceeding to CT scan, in view of minimising the risk of contrast induced nephropathy.
- Urinalysis – remember that haematuria can occur in any renal tract problem, but also can occur in AAA.
- CT with IV contrast –this should clarify a diagnosis – it can identify aortic aneurysms,

PATHOLOGY

renal stones as well as other intra-abdominal causes that may be present.

A plain abdominal film is requested. Discuss the findings.

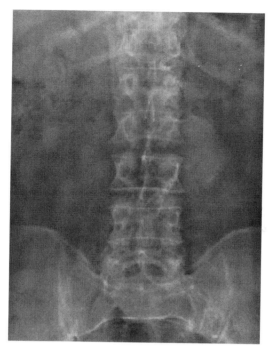

Note the area of calcification in the left paravertebral region – this marks the outline of the wall of the AAA. Calcified arterial vasculature is also a sign of more generalised atherosclerosis.

The patient becomes hypotensive, tachycardic and less responsive (V on AVPU). How can levels of blood loss be classified?

ATLS classification of the stages of haemorrhagic shock:

	I	II	III	IV
Blood loss (ml)	Up to 750	750-1500	1500-2000	>2000
Blood loss (% volume)	<15	15-30	30-40	>40
Pulse rate (bpm)	<100	100-120	120-140	>140
Blood pressure	Normal	Normal	Decreased	Decreased
Pulse pressure (mmHg)	Normal or increased	Decreased	Decreased	Decreased

Resp. rate (rpm)	10-20	20-30	30-35	>35
Urine output (ml/min)	>30	20-30	5-15	Negligible
Central nervous system	Slightly anxious	Mildly anxious	Anxious, confused	Confused, drowsy

When using the classification above, several caveats should be kept in mind. The system tends to underestimate the level of bleeding taking place in the following groups:
• Blunted physiological response (seen in the elderly – unable to mount appropriate tachycardia)
• Concurrent medication use which mask true underlying physiology (e.g. beta-blockade restricting tachycardia)
• Autonomic nervous system dysfunction (e.g. diabetes, Parkinson's disease)

Define an aneurysm?

An aneurysm is an abnormal focal dilatation of a blood vessel wall to a size greater than 1.5 times its normal diameter. An abdominal aorta is usually no more than 1.5-2cm in diameter, therefore at 3cm wide, it would be deemed aneurysmal.

What is the difference between a true and false aneurysm?

A true aneurysm involves all three layers of the vessel wall (i.e. intima, media, and adventitia) whereas a false aneurysm (pseudoaneurysm) involves only one layer. A false aneurysm occurs when there is a breach in a single layer of vessel wall, which blood is driven through by the arterial pressure. This blood is contained by the adventitia or surrounding perivascular soft tissue. A direct communication of blood flow exists between the vessel lumen and the aneurysm lumen through the breach in the vessel wall.

List the potential causes of a true aneurysm?

The aetiology of most aneurysms is multifactorial, but involve the disruption of the elasticity and integrity of the normal vessel wall. Identified risk factors are listed below:
• Severe atherosclerotic damage of the vessel wall:
    o Smoking
    o Hypertension
    o Hyperlipidaemia
    o Male gender
    o Diabetes
• Trauma (including repeated puncture in intravenous drug users).
• Infection – tuberculosis, HIV, salmonella. Infective aneurysms are often referred to as mycotic aneurysms, whether the underlying pathology is a fungal infection of not.
• Connective tissue disorders – Marfan's syndrome, Ehlers-Danlos syndrome type IV.

What are the management options for a ruptured abdominal AAA? Does the CT influence manage options available?

Without surgical intervention, ruptured AAA is fatal. The surgical options include open or endovascular repair of the aorta. In an open repair, the aorta is exposed, aortic and iliac clamps are placed and a prosthetic graft is sewn into place, replacing the aneurysmal segment. During an endovascular aortic repair (EVAR), the aortic graft stent is introduced using the Seldinger technique via the femoral (or more rarely the iliac) artery. This lines the aneurysm, diverting blood flow through the endograft itself and encouraging the now redundant aneurysmal sac to thrombose.

PATHOLOGY

CT aortograms are a vital part of management planning. The morphology of the aneurysm can dictate which method is more appropriate. For example, during EVAR it is necessary that the graft has a clear area of normal non-aneurysmal aortic wall either side of the dilatation, on which to "land" each end of the graft stent. If the aneurysm is conical in shape or too close to visceral branches (e.g. renal arteries), open repair may be more suitable.

Describe the branches of the descending aorta.

The descending aorta has five groups of paired branches and four unpaired branches. They are listed in descending order:
• Inferior phrenic arteries - paired arteries arising posteriorly at the level of T12. They supply the diaphragm.
• Coeliac trunk - unpaired artery arising anteriorly at the level of L1. It supplies the "foregut" (liver, stomach, abdominal oesophagus, spleen, the proximal two thirds of the duodenum and the superior pancreas).
• Superior mesenteric artery - unpaired artery arising anteriorly. It arises at the lower level of L1. It supplies the "midgut" (distal third of duodenum, jejunum, ileum, ascending colon and part of the transverse colon).
• Middle suprarenal arteries - paired arteries that arise either side posteriorly at the level of L1. They supply the adrenal glands.
• Renal arteries - paired arteries arising laterally at the level between L1 and L2. They supply the kidneys.
• Gonadal arteries - paired arteries. Arise laterally at the level of L2.
• Inferior mesenteric artery - unpaired artery. Arises anteriorly at the level of L3. It supplies the "hindgut" (large intestine from the splenic flexure to the upper part of the rectum).
• Median sacral artery - unpaired artery. Arises posteriorly at the level of L4. It supplies the coccyx, lumbar vertebrae and sacrum.
• Lumbar arteries - four pairs of lumbar arteries. Arise posteriorly, between the levels of L1 and L4. They supply the abdominal wall and spinal cord.

The patient returns to ITU following open AAA repair. Later, you are asked to review him regarding complaints of increasing abdominal discomfort and several episodes of dark PR bleed. What do you think may be going on?

It is likely that the patient has ischaemic colitis. Any reduction in blood flow to the bowel wall mucosa can result in ischaemic colitis, and a ruptured AAA presents several mechanisms via which this can happen:
• Global hypoperfusion – secondary to blood loss, low cardiac output
• Focal hypoperfusion – splanchnic circulation vasoconstriction as part of the physiological response to hypovolaemic shock or use of vasopressors
• Occlusion of the inferior mesenteric artery – external compression (retraction during surgery, haematoma), arthero-embolisation, thrombus.
Incidence of ischaemic colitis following AAA repair is 1-3% (for both open and endovascular repair), but rises to 10% in open repair of a ruptured AAA and with increasing age, operation time longer than 4 hours, prolonged cross-clamping of the aorta, sustained hypoperfusion, use of inotropes and renal impairment.

What other complications can occur following open ruptured AAA repair?

• Early complications
  o Anastomosic leak
  o Graft occlusion – thrombus (can cause ischaemic colitis, acute lower limb ischaemia etc)
  o Renal impairment – secondary to peri-operative hypoperfusion (hypovolae

PATHOLOGY

mia, aortic cross-clamping if supra-renal aneurysm), contrast nephropathy from CT scans
   o Respiratory complications – poor mobility and poor cough secondary to pain from large laparotomy wound
   o Post-operative ileus
• Late complications
   o Wound/graft infection
   o Aorto-enteric fistula (can present as gastrointestinal bleed or graft infection)
   o Sexual dysfunction
   o Incisional hernia

Discuss the screening programme in place in the UK for AAA.

The UK screening programme for AAA was started in 2009. It initially covered just England, but now encompasses all countries in the UK. All men aged 65 are invited, while all men older than 65 before commencement of the screening programme are able to self-refer. Participants receive an abdominal ultrasound scan. If an abdominal aortic aneurysm is identified, the patient will be referred for surveillance. Small aneurysms (3-4.5cm) undergo annual ultrasound surveillance to assess for increasing size. Medium-sized aneurysms (4.5-5cm) undergo three-monthly ultrasound assessments. Large aneurysms are referred to a vascular unit for discussion about the need for intervention.

The AAA screening programme aims to reduce the risk of death from ruptured AAA by half through early identification and pre-emptive repair. The risk of having an aneurysm large enough to be at significant risk of rupture is far smaller in men younger than 65 and in women, so these patient groups are not included in the screening programme.

What are the indications for elective AAA repair?

All patients, fit for surgery, with aneurysms of 5.5 cm diameter or greater should be considered for elective surgical repair. The decision regarding surgical intervention is based on the risk of surgery versus rupture for each patient – 5.5cm is deemed the size at which surgical repair is most beneficial, i.e. the risk of rupture is higher than the risk of mortality/significant morbidity from surgery, as per studies such as UKSAT.
In general, the risk of rupture is determined by the aneurysm diameter but rupture rates are higher in patients who smoke, in females, in those with hypertension and in those with a strong family history. Other indications for surgery are rapid expansion (>1cm per year), distal embolisation or onset of worrying symptoms/signs such as back or abdominal pain. Surgery for smaller aneurysms may be indicated if they meet any of these criteria.

SUMMARY

A ruptured AAA may present with sudden-onset abdominal, back or loin pain, usually associated with hypovolaemic shock. Immediate management is centred on gaining IV access, judicious fluid resuscitation and repair of the aorta, whether this by via open surgery or endovascular stent placement

PATHOLOGY

TOP TIPS

➕ Always think about a ruptured AAA in an older patient with new back or loin pain. This is a very common exam scenario and represents a differential diagnosis that needs to be ruled out quickly, before other diagnoses can be assumed. Ruptured AAA can present with haematuria – never assume renal colic in older patients with no history of renal calculi! This is a common pitfall.

➕ Permissive hypotension is an important concept in the management of major haemorrhage such as ruptured AAA – it is a fine balance between ensuring adequate tissue perfusion and avoiding driving further haemorrhage.

➕ Treatment for ruptured AAA requires surgery. This can be open or endovascular – this choice is guided by various factors including aneurysmal morphology, patient fitness for surgery and patient choice

PATHOLOGY

2.10 Inflammatory Bowel Disease

Scenario

You are the surgical CT2. You have been asked to assess a 27 year-old female who presents with a 1 week history of right iliac fossa pain as well as passing blood and mucus per rectum. She has lost 2 stones in weight recently. She does not have a history of recent travel. On further questioning, she mentions that she has a family history of Crohn's disease.

On examination, she is tender and mildly guarding in the right iliac fossa.

What is your differential diagnosis?

- Inflammatory bowel disease
- Infective colitis
- Appendicitis
- Familial adenomatous polyposis
- Ovarian cyst
- Pelvic inflammatory disease

How would you manage this patient?

The patient should be initially assessed and managed in accordance with the CCRiSP protocol, with an ABCDE assessment focussed on identifying and correcting any physiological abnormalities. Pertinent to this scenario is the potential for hypovolaemia, which may necessitate intravenous fluid resuscitation. I would also ensure the patient received appropriate analgesia.

What investigations would aid your diagnosis?

- Bloods (FBC, U&E, LFT, CRP, ESR)
- Stool sample to rule out infective colitis
- MRI can be used to assess extent of disease
- Colonoscopy +/- biopsies

What are the macroscopic differences between ulcerative colitis and Crohn's disease?

	Ulcerative colitis	Crohn's Disease
Distribution	Colon and rectum Rarely terminal ileum Continuous distribution	Whole GI tract. Rectum usually spared. Commonly affects terminal ileum 'Skip' lesions (inflammation is not continous)
Other Features		Pseudopolyp formation 'Cobblestone' appearance
Anal disease	Rare	Perianal skin involvement
Intestinal fistula	Rare	Common
Strictures	Rare	Common

What are the microscopic differences between ulcerative colitis and Crohn's disease?

Ulcerative colitis	Crohn's Disease
Inflammatory changes usually only present in the mucosa	Full thickness (transmural inflammation) leading to cobblestone appearance
No granuloma formation	Non-caseating granulomas
Fissure formation is rare	Fissures are common
Crypt abscesses common	No crypt abscesses

What are the associated extra-alimentary manifestations of inflammatory bowel disease?

Musculoskeletal
• Arthritis (e.g. ankylosing spondylitis, sacroiliitis)
• Hypertrophic osteoarthropathy (e.g. clubbing, periostitis)
• Osteoporosis
• Aseptic necrosis (avascular necrosis)
• Polymyositis

Skin
• Erythema nodosum
• Pyoderma gangrenosum
• Apthous ulcers
• Glossitis
• Purpura
• Hair loss

Hepatopancreatobiliary
• Primary sclerosing cholangitis
• Bile duct carcinoma (cholangiocarcinoma)
• Autoimmune chronic active hepatitis
• Pericholangitis
• Portal fibrosis
• Cirrhosis
• Granulomatous disease
• Fatty liver disease
• Gallstones

Eyes
• Uveitis/iritis
• Episcleritis
• Corneal ulcers
• Retinal vascular disease
• Scleromalacia

Metabolic
• Growth retardation in children
Renal
• Renal stones (calcium oxalate stone deposition)

How would you assess the severity index for ulcerative colitis?

This is based on the Truelove and Witts Criteria.

	Mild	Moderate	Severe
Bowel movements per day	<4	4 – 6	>6 with at least one of the features of systemic upset marked * below
Blood in stools	No more than small amounts of blood	Between mild and severe	Visible blood
Pyrexia (temperature > 37.8oC)*	No	No	Yes
Heart rate > 90 bpm*	No	No	Yes
Anaemia*	No	No	Yes
Erythrocyte sedimentation rate (mm/hour)*	< 30	<30	>30

What are the complications of inflammatory bowel disease (IBD)?

Ulcerative colitis:
- Toxic megacolon
- Bowel obstruction
- Perforation

Crohn's disease:
- Stricture
- Fistula formation
- Abscesses
- Obstruction
- Perforation

How would you manage a patient with IBD?

This is divided into:
1. Managing the acute flare. The goal of therapy is to induce and maintain remission. An acute flare is usually managed with steroids, and remission induced using immunosuppressive therapies including aminosalicylates (5-ASA), azathioprine, methotrexate, or biological agents such as infliximab.

2. Management of complications. This includes maximising medical therapy and supporting nutrition in the first instance. Surgery has a role, and the strategy differs between ulcerative colitis (wherein colectomy has traditionally been considered definitive management) and Chron's (where further surgery is likely and minimal resections are performed in order to preserve bowel length).

What are the indications for surgery for patients presenting with IBD?

- Disease refractory to medical therapy.
- Complications of Crohn's (e.g. fistulating disease, strictures)
- Obstruction
- Perforation

SUMMARY

Inflammatory bowel disease has a complex pathophysiology, with genetic, immunoregulatory and even environmental factors involved in its pathogenesis. Recent research has also implicated commensal bacteria as potential precipitants. The aim of managing inflammatory bowel disease is to induce and maintain remission with as few side effects and medication burden as possible. An important part of management is lifestyle advice, such as smoking cessation.

TOP TIPS

➕ Distinguishing between Crohn's disease and ulcerative colitis is not always easy. This has led many authors to recognise a subtype of IBD- 'indeterminate colitis'.

➕ The differing pathological features of Crohn's and ulcerative colitis lends itself well to an exam question and is well worth becoming familiar with.

➕ Patients with IBD that present with acute abdomen should be thoroughly investigated to assess for complications of IBD, rather that assuming that their presentation is simply a 'flare' of their condition. Similarly, their presentation may not be linked to their condition at all- for example an appendicitis.

PATHOLOGY

2.11 Colorectal Cancer

Scenario

A 72 year-old male presents to the colorectal clinic with a 2 month history of PR bleeding, altered bowel habits and unintentional weight lost of 2 stones over the last 6 months.

On examination, he is cachectic and his abdomen is soft and non-tender. PR examination shows dark red blood mixed with stool.

What is your differential diagnosis?

- Colorectal cancer
- Diverticular disease
- Inflammatory bowel disease
- Haemorrhoids/Anal fissures

How would you manage this patient?

Though in an outpatient setting, the patient should be comprehensively assessed with an A through E approach to ensure that they are stable. In this scenario, there is the possibility of both hypovolemia and symptomatic anaemia which could warrant admission for rehydration/transfusion. Only if there is no need for acute inpatient management can the patient be safely treated as an outpatient.

What investigation would aid your diagnosis?

- Colonoscopy and biopsy (under the 2 week rule)
- Staging CT chest/abdomen/pelvis

What are the risk factors for colorectal cancer?

- Age (≥ 60 years old)
- Diet (high red meat and low fibre)
- High alcohol intake
- Smoking
- History of polyps / colorectal cancer
- Past medical history of inflammatory bowel disease
- Family history of colorectal cancer

What types of colorectal polyps are you aware of?

- **Benign:** juvenile polyps, Peutz-Jeghers syndrome (hamartomatous polyps), metaplastic polyps, adenomas
- **Malignant:** Colorectal carcinoma

What do you understand by the adenoma carcinoma sequence?

This is the stepwise progression of normal epithelial tissue through dysplasia to carcinoma formation. It occurs due to the accumulation of mutations causing activation of oncogenes and inactivation of tumour suppressor genes.

How would you risk-stratify benign colorectal polyps at colonoscopy, and what would be the further management of each strata?

• Low risk – 1-2 adenomas both less than 1cm in size. No surveillance or repeat colonoscopy at 5 years.
• Intermediate risk – 3-4 small adenomas or at least one greater than 1cm. Repeat colonoscopy at 3 years.
• High risk – greater than 5 small adenomas or greater than 3, at least one more than 1cm. Repeat colonoscopy in 1 year.

What is the difference between staging and grading?

Staging is the extent of spread of the disease, and informs on the local invasion of the neoplastic process and also any metastatic disease or lymphatic involvement. Grading refers to a histological finding. It is the degree of differentiation of the diseased tissue, with a lower grade more closely resembling the tissue of origin.

What are the colorectal cancer staging systems?
• Dukes staging

Dukes A	Confined to mucosa
Dukes B	Through the muscularis mucosa
Dukes C	Involvement of one local lymph node
Dukes D	Distant metastasis (e.g. to liver or lungs)

• TNM staging
TNM- standing for tumour, nodes, metastasis- is a staging system which has been adopted for several cancer types. It gives a numeric code for the local extent of disease (T), the number of involved lymph nodes (N), and the site and number of distant metastasis (M).

Name and summarise any clinical syndromes associated with colorectal tumours.

• Familial adenomatous polyposis (FAP)
 o Autosomal dominant inheritance
 o Associated with loss of the APC tumour suppressor gene on Chromosome 5
 o Associated with a 100% risk of cancer
 o Most patients develop colorectal cancer by age 40s
 o Patients have greater than 100 polyps in the colon on colonoscopy
 o Patients with FAP also have a higher risk of upper GI cancer and therefore upper GI endoscopic surveillance is recommended
 o FAP is also associated with small bowel polyps and mandibular osteoma (known as Gardner Syndrome)
 o Most patients will be offered prophylactic colectomy with regular stump surveillance

• Hereditary Non-polyposis Colorectal Cancer (HNPCC) also known as Lynch Syndrome
 o Autosomal dominant inheritance with a strong family history.
 o Comprises 2-5% of all colorectal cancers
 o Associated with DNA repair gene mutation (mhl1 and msh2)
 o Early presentation with increased risk of developing endometrial/ovarian/gastric and other cancers
 o 70-80% lifetime risk of developing colorectal cancer

• Peutz-Jeghers Syndrome
 o Multiple hamartomatous polyps throughout the GI tract
 o Low malignant potential

PATHOLOGY

SUMMARY

Colorectal cancer is the third most common cancer in the UK in both men and women. The majority arise through the adenoma-carcinoma sequence, initially forming as an adenomatous polyp and becoming malignant as clonally-expanded mutations accumulate. There are three main histological subtypes of colonic adenoma: tubular, tubulovillous, and villous. Of the three, villous adenomas have the greatest malignant potential. In the UK, the bowel cancer screening program involves a postal faecal-occult-blood test. It is sent to people between the ages of 60 and 74 every two years.

TOP TIPS

 Guidelines on the surveillance and management of colorectal cancer are available from the British Society of Gastroenterology.

2.12 | Fistulae

Scenario

A 64-year-old lady with known diverticular disease has been referred to you by her GP as she has been complaining of a 4-month history of recurrent urinary tract infections and passing faeculent material in her urine.

What is your differential diagnosis?

Urinary tract infection (recurrent/treatment-resistant)
Colovesical fistula
Other fistula (e.g. colovaginal)

How would you investigate this patient?

• CT abdomen/pelvis- can confirm the presence of a fistula and delineate the anatomy if present. Will also inform on the extent of the diverticular disease
• Colonoscopy- can assess the presence and extent of diverticular disease and identify other causes for symptoms.
• Flexible cystoscopy- can confirm the presence of a fistula and may identify any other cause for the symptoms

Investigations confirm the presence of a colovesical fistula. How would you manage this patient?

• The recurrent urinary tract infections should be managed with an extended course of antibiotics guided by urinary MC&S, with advice from microbiology if required
• Defunctioning loop colostomy can be used to divert faeces and prevent recurrent UTI
• Colonic resection, primary anastomosis and bladder repair is likely the definitive management. This could be performed either laparoscopically or as an open procedure

What is the definition of a fistula?

A fistula is an abnormal communication between two epithelialised surfaces.

How does a fistula differ to a sinus?

A sinus is a blind-ending tract lined with epithelial cells, as opposed to an open tract between surfaces (e.g. hollow organ to skin or between two hollow organs)

How would you manage a patient with fistula?

Patients with fistulae may present differently depending on the site of the fistula. For example, those with fistula-in-ano can be successfully managed in the outpatient setting. However, fistulas can become a significant source of morbidity leading to sepsis and/or malnutrition. The mnemonic 'SNAP' can be used as a tool to plan management:

• Sepsis – investigate for signs of sepsis and treat aggressively if present
• Nutrition – assess for any nutritional deficit and provide supplements/involve a dietician if necessary. In some circumstances it may even be necessary to consider total parenteral nutrition (TPN)
• Assess the anatomy- clearly understanding the anatomy of the fistulous tract is important. CT is the initial modality of choice, though further imaging such as MRI may have a

PATHOLOGY

role
• Plan surgery- though many fistulas will heal with conservative management and the steps outlined above

What factors affect fistula formation?

Again, these factors can be recalled with a mnemonic: FRIENDS.
• Foreign body
• Radiation
• Iatrogenic/Infection/Inflammatory
• Epithelialisation
• Neoplasia
• Distal obstruction
• Short tract (<2cm)

What are the other complications of diverticular disease?

• Diverticulitis
• Diverticular abscess
• Diverticular mass
• Bleeding
• Perforation
• Fistula (as in this case)

What are the complications of TPN?

Complications can be considered as related to the insertion or maintenance of the central line, and those related to the TPN itself.

Related to catheter insertion:
• Arterial puncture
• Pneumothorax
• Haemothorax
• Arrhythmia
• Cardiac tamponade

Line related complications:
• Line blockage
• Sepsis

TPN related complications:
• Hyperglycaemia
• Refeeding syndrome
• Fluid overload
• Liver failure
• Renal failure

SUMMARY

The key management of fistulae is to treat the underlying pathology and reduce fistula output using the SNAP mnemonic. The majority of fistulae will heal with conservative management therefore avoiding the need for surgery. This scenario has focussed on GI fistulae, but it is important to bear in mind that fistulae can form between any two epithelialised surfaces. For example, labyrinthine fistulae can present with imbalance or difficulty hearing.

TOP TIPS

 Remember not all fistulae are pathological. For example, arteriovenous fistulae can be formed surgically to facilitate dialysis.

PATHOLOGY

2.13 Appendicitis

Scenario

You are the surgical CT2 on-call and have been referred a 17 year-old female with sudden onset paraumbilical pain radiating to the right iliac fossa. She does not have any urinary symptoms. Her last menstrual period was 2 weeks ago.
Her observations are as follows: HR 110, BP130/90, Temp 37.9oC, O2 sats 98% on air
On examination, she is tender and guarding in the right iliac fossa.

What is your differential diagnosis?

- Appendicitis
- Mesenteric adenitis
- Ectopic pregnancy
- Inflammatory bowel disease
- Ovarian cyst
- Mittelschmerz
- Meckel's diverticulitis
- Pelvic inflammatory disease
- Urinary tract infection

How would you manage this patient?

This patient should initially be assessed using the ABCDE algorithm. IV access should be gained and any physiological abnormalities identified and corrected. Blood tests should be taken and sent, and urine collected for urinalysis and pregnancy testing. IV fluids should be commenced and the patient kept nil by mouth. An erect chest radiograph should be performed. The on-call surgical registrar or consultant should be notified, and (depending on clinical suspicion) the emergency theatre and anaesthetic teams should be notified.

What is the common pathophysiology of appendicitis?

Appendicitis is most often caused by obstruction of the lumen by faecoliths. The lumen distal to the obstruction starts to fill with mucus, leading to increased intraluminal and intramural pressures and an increase in the number of bacteria present. Over time, the small venules and capillaries become thrombosed leading to engorgement and venocongestion. An acute inflammatory response is initiated. Ultimately, the appendix becomes ischaemic, leading to infarction and perforation.

Describe the blood supply of the appendix

The appendix is supplied by the appendicular artery which is a branch of the ileocolic artery. This runs in the mesoappendix adjacent to the appendicular wall. Venous drainage occurs via the ileocolic veins and the right colic vein into the portal vein.

Describe the possible locations of the appendix

Though the base of the appendix has a relatively constant location at the convergence of the taeniae coli, there is no fixed position of the body and tip. The appendix can therefore be described as retroperitoneal, pelvic, pre- or post-ileal (in front of or behind the terminal ileum), retrocaecal (behind the caecum), or even beside or beneath the ascending colon or liver.

List the common complications of appendicitis

- Sepsis
- Perforation
- Peritonitis
- Abscess formation

What are the available surgical options for performing an appendicectomy?

Appendicectomy can be performed either laparoscopically or as an open procedure. In modern practice, laparoscopic appendicectomy is the norm in uncomplicated cases.

What types of incisions would you perform in an open appendicectomy?

The gridiron or Lanz incisions are the most commonly used for open appendicectomy. The gridiron incision, or McBurney's incision, is centred over McBurney's point. It is an oblique incision at a right angle to the line running between the anterior superior iliac spine and the umbilicus (the incision therefore runs from superolateral to inferomedial). The Lanz incision is a modification resulting in a more transverse incision with improved cosmesis. The centre of the incision is the same, but the line of the incision is along Langer's line.

Describe the layers traversed when performing an open appendicectomy

- Skin
- Subcutaneous fat
- Fascia (Camper and Scarpa's layers)
- External oblique aponeurosis
- Internal oblique
- Transversus abdominis
- Pre-peritoneal fat
- Peritoneum

The patient has been diagnosed with appendicitis and you have been asked to consent her for theatre. What are the potential complications you would counsel her about?

General complications:
- Pain
- Bleeding
- Scarring
- Damage to surrounding structures
- DVT/PE risk
- Incisional hernia

Specific to laparoscopic appendicectomy:
- Bloating
- Bowel injury
- Port site herniation
- Increased risk of fetal loss (if pregnant) than in open surgery
- Conversion to open surgery

PATHOLOGY

SUMMARY

Appendicitis is the most common general surgical emergency with an annual incidence of approximately 10 cases per 100,000 of the population. It is thought to be associated with dietary habits and a lower intake of dietary fibre. The classical presentation is the onset of vague paraumbilical pain which becomes localised to the right iliac fossa as the inflamed appendix begins to irritate the parietal peritoneum.

TOP TIPS

 Many surgeons advocate 'running' the small bowel at the time of appendicectomy, looking for the presence of a Meckel's diverticulum, as Meckel's diverticulitis can mimic appendicitis.

PATHOLOGY

2.14 Jaundice

Scenario

You are the surgical CT2 on-call and have been referred a 33 year-old lady who presents with right upper quadrant pain and vomiting. During the history, she admits to having noticed dark urine and pale stools.
Her observations are as follows: HR 120, BP 105/65, Temp 38.5oC, O2 sats 96% on air.

What is your differential diagnosis?

- Acute cholecystitis
- Ascending cholangitis
- Choledocholithiasis
- Biliary colic
- Pancreatic adenocarcinoma

How would you initially manage this patient?

Initial assessment of this patient should be with the ABCDE protocol, identifying and correcting haemodynamic abnormalities whilst ensuring adequate IV access. This patient is septic and should be treated in accordance with 'the Sepsis 6'. Blood cultures and lactate should be sent and accurate fluid balance monitoring established. Intravenous antibiotics, oxygen therapy and intravenous resuscitation should be commenced. The most likely cause of sepsis in this case is biliary, and therefore the appropriate antibiotics for intra-abdominal sepsis in accordance with local protocol should be commenced.

What investigations would aid your diagnosis?

- Ultrasound- ultrasonography to assess the appearance of the gallbladder and biliary tree and look for the presence (and location) of gallstones
- Magnetic resonance cholangiopancreatography (MRCP)- can further assess the biliary tree if the diagnosis remains uncertain
- Endoscopic retrograde cholangiopancreatography (ERCP)- in addition to aiding diagnosis, ERCP also offers the possibility of therapeutic biliary sphincterotomy and stenting and stone extraction

What are the complications of gallstone disease?

Within the gallbladder
- acute cholecystitis
- biliary colic
- empyema
- Mirizzi's syndrome

Within the common bile duct
- ascending cholangitis
- obstructive jaundice

In the pancreas
- acute pancreatitis

PATHOLOGY

Within the bowel
• gallstone ileus

What are the complications of ERCP?

• Pain
• Bleeding
• Perforation
• Acute pancreatitis
• Failure of procedure/equipment
• Biliary reflux following sphincterotomy

Describe the production and metabolism of bilirubin

• Production is initiated in the reticuloendothelial system
• Haem-oxygenase enzymes break down haem, removing iron and carbon monoxide to leave biliverdin
• Biliverdin is then converted into bilirubin by the enzyme biliverdin reductase
• Bilirubin (unconjugated) then enters the circulation, and is later removed from the circulation in the liver by the sinusoidal hepatocytes
• Bilirubin 'conjugated' through being bound to glucuronic acid by glucuronyl transferase

How can jaundice be classified?

Jaundice can be considered as pre-hepatic, hepatic, or post-hepatic.

Pre-hepatic
• Increased bilirubin (increased haem turnover)
• Decreased transport to the liver

Hepatic
• Defective uptake of bilirubin
• Defective conjugation
• Defective excretion of bilirubin by liver cells

Post-hepatic
• Defective transport of bilirubin by the biliary duct system

Give some examples of the causes of jaundice

Pre-hepatic
• Hereditary spherocytosis
• Haemolytic anaemia
• Pernicious anaemia
• Incompatible blood transfusion

Hepatic
• Hepatitis
• Cirrhosis
• Drugs
• Toxins
• Gilbert's syndrome
• Liver tumours (primary or secondary)

Post-hepatic
• Intraluminal obstruction e.g.: gallstones
• Obstruction in the wall of the biliary tree e.g. biliary atresia, stricture, chronic cholangitis,

cholangiocarcinoma
• External compression e.g.: pancreatitis, tumour, pancreatic cyst formation.

SUMMARY

Ultrasound scans are more sensitive at detecting the presence of stones within the gall-bladder rather than the common bile duct (CBD). They can, however, measure the calibre of the CBD and thus prompt further investigation with MRCP or ERCP. The calibre of CBD considered normal is 4mm in an adult patient aged 40 or less. The acceptable calibre increases by 1mm every decade thereafter. For example, a 7mm CBD in a 70-year-old patient may be normal, but would be abnormal in a 30 year old patient.

BSG guidelines advocate ERCP within 48 hours in patients who fall into the following categories:

1. Predicted or actual severe pancreatitis
2. Ascending cholangitis
3. Unresolving jaundice
4. Dilated CBD

TOP TIPS

 An important *(and sometimes overlooked)* part of the management of biliary colic is a strict fat-free diet.

PATHOLOGY

2.15 | Bone Healing

Scenario

You are on call for Orthopaedics and the emergency department registrar asks you to review a radiograph taken of a 30-year-old's ankle. She sustained this injury when she fell down two steps. The injury is closed, isolated and distally neurovascular intact.

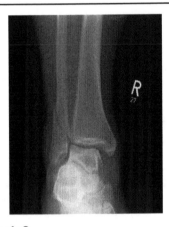

What is your diagnosis?

There is a Weber B fracture of the right fibula with associated talar shift.

How would you manage this patient?

All assessments in the emergency setting should begin with ensuring the patient is stable and not in need of any resuscitation. In this situation, it is an isolated injury in an otherwise well patient. A comprehensive history and examination should be performed, in particular assessing the neurovascular status of the limb distal to the injury. Adequate, appropriate analgesia should be administered to allow reduction of the fracture and initial stabilisation in a below-knee back slab. After any manipulation or plaster application, the injury should be re-imaged and the neurovascular status reassessed. At this point, the case should be discussed with the appropriate orthopaedic seniors with a view to potentially arranging fixation in theatre.

What investigation would aid your diagnosis

Orthogonal radiographs (AP and lateral) and a mortise view of the ankle. If there is any more proximal (or distal) tenderness the relevant radiographs should be taken and reviewed. As a general rule of thumb, images should be obtained of the joint above and below. In this scenario, a post-manipulation/plaster radiograph should also be obtained.

As this is an injury potentially requiring open reduction and internal fixation, an assessment of the patients' anaesthetic fitness should be performed. This may include an ECG, routine biochemistry, clotting studies, and any other investigations suggested by the history.

What are the principal stages of fracture healing?

Bone healing can be separated into 4 principal stages:

Inflammation: this stage begins almost immediately and persists for approximately a week. Haematoma forms at the fracture site, and local inflammation occurs with migration of inflammatory cells and a cascade of pro-inflammatory mediators. Necrotic bone at the fracture site is removed by osteoclasts, and the haematoma is gradually replaced by granulation tissue.

Soft callus: follows from the inflammatory stage. This is the formation of calcified fibrocartilage across the fracture site.

Hard callus: occurs with recruitment of osteoblast precursors and angiogenesis into the bridging soft callus. The tissue is ossified into woven bone.

Remodelling: occurs over the course of months or years after the fracture. The woven bone across the fracture site is remodelled into dense lamellar bone. This remodelling occurs in relation to the stresses experienced by the bone (Wolff's law).

Explain the difference between primary and secondary bone healing

Primary bone healing only occurs in situations of anatomic reduction and absolute stability. There is angiogenesis across any (very) small gaps, with the recruitment of osteoblast precursors. 'Cutting cones' form with osteoclasts at the head and traverse the fracture site, allowing angiogenesis and the laying down of lamellar bone in their wake. There is no callus formation- this is the process involved in the remodelling phase described above.

Secondary bone healing is achieved with relative stability, and follows the stages described previously with callus formation.

What are delayed union, non-union and malunion?

Delayed union occurs when there is a delay in fracture healing beyond that which is expected for a particular fracture. If a delayed union fails to heal, then it becomes a non-union. If the fracture unites, but in an improper position, this is termed a malunion.

How can non-union be classified?

Non-union can be subdivided into hypertrophic or atrophic non-union. Hypertrophic non-union is usually due to excess mobility at the fracture site. This prevents the ossification and remodelling of callus into bone. Atrophic non-union usually occurs secondary to poor blood supply (e.g. from excessive stripping of the periosteum).

List some risk factors for delayed union/malunion/ non-union?

Smoking
Increased age
Infection
Ischaemia (e.g. poor peripheral blood supply)
Increased interfragmentary strain (inadequate immobilisation)
Interposition of tissue between the fragments
Severe local trauma
Bone loss
Malnutrition (e.g. vitamin d deficiency)
Metabolic bone disease

PATHOLOGY

Osteoporosis

What is Perren's strain theory?

Perren's strain theory relates to fracture healing. Cellular activity at a fracture site seems to be related to the degree of strain across that fracture site. Decreasing strain stimulates the formation of (in order of decreasing strain): granulation tissue to connective tissue to fibrocartilage to bone. For example, in relative stability there is movement (and therefore strain) at the fracture site stimulating the formation of connective tissue callus, which reduces the strain and allows progression to hard callus. This further reduces strain, later favouring bone formation.

What is a Haversian canal?

The Haversian canals are the central neurovascular channel within an osteon of cortical bone. They communicate with adjacent Haversian systems via Volkmann canals.

What is CRPS?

CRPS stands for complex regional pain syndrome type 1, also known as Sudek's atrophy. It involves a complex disorder of pain, sensory abnormalities, abnormal blood flow, autonomic symptoms, and trophic changes in superficial or deep tissues without evidence of nerve injury. It can be caused by traumatic or surgical injury, herpes zoster, myocardial infarction or can be idiopathic.

Patients usually present weeks to months after an initial injury with lancing pain, hyperalgesia or allodynia in a neighbouring area to the initial injury. They may also have vasomotor symptoms and the skin can be swollen or trophic and shiny. Other neuromuscular symptoms include weakness, hyperreflexia, dystonia and contractures. It is usually self-limiting. However, management should involve referral to the pain team, and use of treatments such as amitriptyline, gabapentin or sympathetic nerve blocks.

SUMMARY

Bone healing occurs in a predictable sequence and is an important topic for a number of reasons. Firstly, problems with bone healing leading to delayed/non-union are a significant source of morbidity. Bone healing can be affected by local (e.g. adequacy of immobilisation at the fracture site) and systemic (e.g. smoking) factors. It is also important as it underpins fracture fixation: absolute stability preventing strain at the fracture site and therefore facilitating primary bone healing (e.g. ORIF) versus relative stability allowing slight movement at the fracture site to stimulate callus formation (e.g. IM fixation).

TOP TIPS

 Secondary bone healing occurs with callus formation, primary occurs without. Thus primary will usually only occur with anatomical, rigid fixation.

PATHOLOGY

21776213R00071

Printed in Great Britain
by Amazon